Silvan Urfer

Lifespan and Causes of Death in the Irish Wolfhound

Silvan Urfer

Lifespan and Causes of Death in the Irish Wolfhound

Medical, Genetical and Ethical Aspects

Südwestdeutscher Verlag für Hochschulschriften

Impressum / Imprint
Bibliografische Information der Deutschen Nationalbibliothek: Die Deutsche Nationalbibliothek verzeichnet diese Publikation in der Deutschen Nationalbibliografie; detaillierte bibliografische Daten sind im Internet über http://dnb.d-nb.de abrufbar.
Alle in diesem Buch genannten Marken und Produktnamen unterliegen warenzeichen-, marken- oder patentrechtlichem Schutz bzw. sind Warenzeichen oder eingetragene Warenzeichen der jeweiligen Inhaber. Die Wiedergabe von Marken, Produktnamen, Gebrauchsnamen, Handelsnamen, Warenbezeichnungen u.s.w. in diesem Werk berechtigt auch ohne besondere Kennzeichnung nicht zu der Annahme, dass solche Namen im Sinne der Warenzeichen- und Markenschutzgesetzgebung als frei zu betrachten wären und daher von jedermann benutzt werden dürften.

Bibliographic information published by the Deutsche Nationalbibliothek: The Deutsche Nationalbibliothek lists this publication in the Deutsche Nationalbibliografie; detailed bibliographic data are available in the Internet at http://dnb.d-nb.de.
Any brand names and product names mentioned in this book are subject to trademark, brand or patent protection and are trademarks or registered trademarks of their respective holders. The use of brand names, product names, common names, trade names, product descriptions etc. even without a particular marking in this works is in no way to be construed to mean that such names may be regarded as unrestricted in respect of trademark and brand protection legislation and could thus be used by anyone.

Verlag / Publisher:
Südwestdeutscher Verlag für Hochschulschriften
ist ein Imprint der / is a trademark of
AV Akademikerverlag GmbH & Co. KG
Heinrich-Böcking-Str. 6-8, 66121 Saarbrücken, Deutschland / Germany
Email: info@svh-verlag.de

Herstellung: siehe letzte Seite /
Printed at: see last page
ISBN: 978-3-8381-0585-7

Zugl. / Approved by: Bern, Universität Bern, Inaugural-Dissertation, 2007

Copyright © 2009 AV Akademikerverlag GmbH & Co. KG
Alle Rechte vorbehalten. / All rights reserved. Saarbrücken 2009

Omnia mors poscit – lex est, non poena perire

(Seneca)

For Garbhan, Nancy, Gail, Peter, Ebony, George, Jack, Max, Graham, Gillian, Fionna, Granua, Thomas, Victor, Iontac, Lolo, Nanna, Donaghue and all the others

Table of Contents

Acknowledgements iv
1 Introduction 1
   1.1 First Edition 1
   1.2 Second Edition 3
2 Abstract/Summary 5
   2.1 Literature Review (chapter 3) 5
   2.2 Lifespan, Causes of Death, Genetics (chapters 4 to 6) 6
   2.3 Discussion and Conclusions (chapter 7) 8
3 Literature Review 11
   3.1 Lifespan in General 11
   3.2 Intrahepatic Portosystemic Shunt (PSS) 17
   3.3 Dilatative Cardiomyopathy (DCM) 21
   3.4 Osteogenic Sarcoma (OS) 27
   3.5 Gastric Dilation and Volvulus (GDV) 31
   3.6 Rhinitis/Bronchopneumonia Syndrome – PCD 35
   3.7 Juvenile Fibrocartilaginous Embolism (FCE) 37
   3.8 Epilepsy 41
   3.9 Osteochondrosis (OC) 45
   3.10 Von Willebrand's Disease (vWD) 48
   3.11 Progressive Retinal Atrophy (PRA) 50
   3.12 Miscellaneous 52
   3.13 Clinical Reference Values 56
4 Dogs, Materials and Methods 59
   4.1 Dogs 59
   4.2 Software 59
   4.3 Definition of Causes of Death 61
   4.4 Definition of Right Censored Data 61
5 Results of Past Studies Revisited 62
   5.1 Re-analysis of Bernardi (1986) and Prokopenko (1998) 62
   5.2 Analysis of Murphy (1991) 66
6 Analysis of the Present Data 71
   6.1 Population Structure and Genetics 71
   6.2 Lifespan 75
   6.3 Population Genetics of Dogs Born 1965 and After 83
   6.4 Ancestor Analyses of Diseases Presumed Hereditary 88
7 Discussion 98
   7.1 Lifespan 98
   7.2 Population Genetics 103
   7.3 Ethical Considerations 112
   7.4 Future Prospects in Breeding 117
   7.5 Future Research Prospects 120
8 References 123
9 Appendix 133

Acknowledgements

The author wishes to thank the following persons and institutions, without whose help and support this study would not have been possible:

Prof. Dr. Andreas Steiger for the overall supervision

Prof. em. Dr. Claude Gaillard for his enthousiastic help with the genetic analyses

Mrs. M.A. André, BS, for making her pedigree database available

Colonel Martin Ruch, DVM, for his general help and support, and the Veterinary Competence Centre of the Swiss Army for its financial support

Mrs. Gretchen Bernardi and Dr. Susan Prokopenko for making their respective lifespan study data available

Mrs. Laurie Bingaman-Lackey of the International Species Information System (ISIS) for her help with the pedigree charts

Ms. E.C. Murphy for taking the effort of collecting and publishing an extensive lifespan database (Murphy 1991)

Ms. A.I. Gottsch for filling in various gaps in the pedigree information

The Small Animal Clinics of the Vetsuisse Faculty in Berne and Zurich for the health information from their clinical databases

Various university researchers throughout the world for their comments and for making their study data available

Various breeders and owners, Swiss and foreign, for submitting health data of their Wolfhounds

Prof. Dr. Irene Sommerfeld-Stur of the Veterinary University of Vienna; Sabine Gebhardt-Hendrich, PhD, Andrina Hauzenberger, DVM, Patrizia Eberli, MVM, and Jérôme Föllmi, DVM, of the Vetsuisse Faculty of Berne, for their suggestions and critique

And last but not least, all the many people who welcomed me to their houses and kennels over the past six years.

1 Introduction

1.1 First Edition

"It is impossible to understand the present without knowing the past."

The Irish Wolfhound is a breed of dog that has been gaining in popularity considerably over the past three decades (see chapter 6.1.1). As a result, the number of veterinary papers on the subject has been increasing steadily. Thus, it suggested itself to bring some organisation into the work that already exists on the subject, and conducting some original research was added as an integral part of a thesis.

As this study shows, there are a substantial enough number of articles on health conditions in Irish Wolfhounds in the veterinary literature to warrant writing a review article. The goal was to provide interested clinicians with a tool to broaden their knowledge of Irish Wolfhounds as a breed with its specific disease predilections, as well as to enable them to counsel breeders and owners on the modes of inheritance of different diseases and, subsequently, selection against them.

The author has also been frequently confronted with a number of questions on the genetics and lifespan of Irish Wolfhounds in the past, such as:

- Did Irish Wolfhounds live longer in the past than they do nowadays?
- Are there familial and/or geographical differences in lifespan?
- Are there familial and/or geographical differences in the incidence of certain diseases?
- What are the genetic bases of lifespan?
- Are there negative effects of inbreeding in Irish Wolfhounds?
- Can founder animals for certain diseases be identified in the breed history?
- What strategies should be used to improve health and longevity in the breed?

Opinions on these questions vary greatly among different dog fanciers, but rarely are they based on anything but what is referred to as "personal experience" – a person's own subjective impressions, which are not usually based on a significant number of observations, nor on any statistical evaluation thereof, and the value of which is probably as inconsistent as the opinions are themselves. Confirmation bias might also play an important role in the variety of opinions encountered.

This study endeavours to find some responses to these questions that are based on a large amount of data and standardised statistical analysis. While not all of the above questions could be answered satisfactorily, it was possible to shed some light on demographic trends, inbreeding influence, lifespan development over time, founder animals of the modern population and, to a certain degree, geographical, familial and founder influence on lifespan and causes of death through this approach.

When reading veterinary papers on hereditary conditions in dogs in general and Irish Wolfhounds in particular, it is common to find publications that were unable (or unwilling) to track pedigree information of the studied dogs going back more than just a few generations. Putting a pedigree database together from national studbooks and other sources is a time-consuming task that few researchers have the resources to undertake to reach the highest possible number of generations. As a consequence, inaccurate results when calculating genetic parameters such as lowered inbreeding and relationship coefficients are commonplace. Dahlbom, Andersson et al. (1997), Broschk (2004) and Casal, Munuve et al. (2006) are such examples of underestimated inbreeding coefficients in Irish Wolfhounds due to either incomplete pedigrees or an insufficient number of generations considered, and it seems likely that this effect has occurred in numerous genetic studies of other companion animals as well. The importance of as complete pedigrees as possible is also demonstrated through the important differences between 5-, 10- and 20-generation Wright's as well as Meuwissen's inbreeding coefficients found in this study.

Nowadays, a wealth of pedigree information exists on the Internet thanks to the work of dog fanciers who are putting together pedigree databases of their respective breeds, often using quite meticulous methodologies. In future research, this could prove to be an extremely useful source of information for geneticists trying to determine the modes of inheritance of diseases in different dog populations by both saving them the time that would be needed to compile such databases and allowing them to calculate much more accurate genetic parameters for the individuals they are studying.

To the author's knowledge, this study is the first of its kind to use such a privately compiled international pedigree database as a base for an analysis of population genetics and hereditary modes in dogs. Other researches of canine genetics are encouraged to try and find similar databases for the breeds of their interest. They usually represent hundreds, if not thousands of hours of work done by fanciers, many of whom will be very willing to submit their work as a base for scientific research.

The study is divided into the following three parts:

The first part (chapter 3) provides an exhaustive review of the veterinary medical literature published on lifespan and the breed-specific disease predilections that have been reported in Irish Wolfhounds, including information on heredity and current treatment protocols. Additionally, some lay literature on the subject of Wolfhound lifespan is also reviewed.

The second part (chapters 4 to 6) focuses on the analysis of a worldwide pedigree database consisting of 50'822 Irish Wolfhounds born between 1862 and 2005, describing developments in demographics and population genetics over time and their interaction with lifespan and causes of death. Additionally, the population born after 1965 is analysed separately for the same parameters, also including analysis of important ancestors (founders) of the overall population and how ancestors differ between sub-populations affected with different hereditary diseases.

The third part (chapter 7) discusses the findings of the previous chapters and their implications for breeding strategies.

Bern, April 2007

1.2 Second Edition

More than two years have now passed since the first edition of the study at hand was published. Since then, new research on the subject of Irish Wolfhounds has been added to the veterinary literature, which has been incorporated into the second edition:

Researchers in Germany have tried to identify genetic markers for Dilated Cardiomyopathy (DCM), which has so far only resulted in the exclusion of several possible genes as a cause of the disease. A genome-wide association study for the disease in the United States had to be put on hold due to opposition by the Irish Wolfhound Foundation. The results that have been published on DCM have been added to chapter 3.3.

New evidence published by the Utrecht research group in the Netherlands makes it unlikely that portosystemic shunt (PSS) is a simple recessive condition with complete penetrance in Irish Wolfhounds as had been published in the first edition. While the postulated mode of inheritance does not fundamentally alter the breeding recommendations and ethical implications described in the first edition, some changes were necessary in the chapters dealing with the disease.

While no new results have been published in the peer-reviewed literature on the subject of epilepsy, it has been stated by researchers at UPenn that a promising region on chromosome 22 has been identified, which may be linked to the disease in Irish Wolfhounds.

Several case reports on new diseases in the breed have been published since 2007, although none of them seem to indicate the presence of newly emerging breed-specific health problems. The references to these studies have been added to chapter 3.12.

The growth pattern of Irish Wolfhounds as compared to some other large-breed dogs has been studied in Norway. Given the correlation between size and lifespan in the domestic dog, the results of the study have also been added to chapter 3.

As a result of the previous study, the author has published a paper on the problem of right censored data in veterinary lifespan studies (Urfer 2008). The problem seems to be more widespread in the literature than was previously thought, leading to widespread bias in published lifespan estimates in domestic dogs and cats. The paper has been added to the appendix of this book.

There have also been some advances in further researching the lack of inbreeding effects on Irish Wolfhounds, where it could be demonstrated that inbreeding does not seem to have an effect on fertility as far as registered litter size is concerned. The new paper on this subject published by the author (Urfer 2009) has also been added to the appendix.

Seattle, August 2009

2 Abstract/Summary

This study investigates lifespan, causes of death and genetic parameters in the Irish Wolfhound. It is divided into the following three parts:

2.1 Literature Review (chapter 3)

There are an important number of publications dealing with lifespan and disease predispositions in the Irish Wolfhound in the veterinary literature. Published lifespan values vary depending on the study and its publication time. Cohort Bias is defined as a mechanism that artificially lowers the measured lifespan due to right censored data when data are sorted by year of death rather than year of birth.

Irish Wolfhounds are subject to a number of hereditary diseases. Their prevalences and modes of inheritance as published in the literature are summarised in table 1.1

Diseases of Proved Hereditary Origin	Prevalence	Mode of Inheritance
Dilated Cardiomyopathy	12.1% to 27.1%	Mixed monogenic-polygenic; major gene; h^2 = 0.58 to 0.64
Intrahepatic Portosystemic Shunt (patent Ductus venosus)	2.1% to 3.4%; 18% of litters	Autosomal recessive, probably oligogenic (digenic, triallelic)
Rhinitis/Bronchopneumonia (PCD)	Unknown	Probably simple autosomal recessive; reported from six families to-date
Epilepsy	Unknown	Highly heritable (h^2 = 0.87), but genetically complex
Von Willebrand's Disease	High (21%), but of little clinical relevance	Simple autosomal intermediate
Progressive Retinal Atrophy	0.1% (little data available)	Simple autosomal recessive
Diseases with Hereditary Components	**Prevalence**	**Mode of Inheritance**
Osteogenic Sarcoma	21% to 24% (lay data). Odds ratio: 27.5	Complex, with environmental interaction. Familial predisposition described in many breeds including the Deerhound and the St. Bernard.
Gastric Dilation Volvulus	11.5% (lay data) 1.8% to 2.6% (incidence p.a.)	Complex, with environmental interaction. Having an affected relative increases disease risk by 63%
Osteochondrosis	8.9% to 11.8% Odds ratio: 3.5	Polygenic inheritance with environmental interaction. h^2 = 0.25 to 0.45
Juvenile Fibrocartilaginous Embolism (FCE)	Unknown	Possible familial predisposition

Table 1.1: Hereditary diseases in Irish Wolfhounds as reported in the veterinary literature. Odds ratios relate to the prevalence in the overall dog population.

Apart from the diseases mentioned in table 1.1, the veterinary literature includes reports for testosterone-independent low libido and sperm quality, cervical spondylomyelopathy (Wobbler syndrome), posterior cortical cataracts, extraocular myositis and acquired strabismus, calcinosis circumscripta, atypical hepatic encephalopathy following portosystemic shunt, spinal nephroblastoma, juvenile nephropathy, and cricopharyngeal achalasia. Reference values for haematology, growth patterns and blood pressure have also been published.

2.2 Lifespan, Causes of Death, Genetics (chapters 4 to 6)

2.2.1 Right Censored Data ("Cohort Bias")

Lifespan studies published to-date were found to be subject to a phenomenon that we decided to call Cohort Bias: an artificial decrease of measured lifespan if dogs are grouped by year of death rather than year of birth, which is due to right censored data. This bias was removed in the re-analyses and the analysis of our own data, resulting in changes in the results of previously published lifespan studies.

2.2.2 Past Studies

Three previous studies (Bernardi 1986; Murphy 1991; Prokopenko 1998) for which the original data were made available are analysed for lifespan, causes of death and their interactions. Since no significant differences were found between two of the datasets (Bernardi 1986; Prokopenko 1998), these were merged for analysis.

2.2.2.1 Bernardi (1986) and Prokopenko (1998) (n=399)

Mean lifespan was 7.35 ± 2.64 years. The data showed a significantly increased risk of Dilatative Cardiomyopathy in males and a significantly increased risk of cancer other than osteogenic sarcoma in females. Females lived significantly longer than males, and castrated females lived significantly longer than intact females. Castrated males were at a significantly increased risk of osteogenic sarcoma, which was consistent with former studies in dogs. Although their average life expectancy was decreased by six months as compared to intact males, this effect was not significant.

Since these studies did not include sufficient pedigree information, no genetic analyses could be performed.

2.2.2.2 Murphy (1991) (n=336)

Mean lifespan in the Murphy data was 8.75 ± 2.25 years. Females lived significantly longer than males. No information on causes of death and castration status was available. No significant correlations between lifespan and Wright's Inbreeding Coefficients over 5, 10 and 20 generations as well as Meuwissen's Inbreeding Coefficients were found.

2.2.3 Own Data

A worldwide pedigree database consisting of 50'822 Irish Wolfhounds born between 1862 and 2005 was available, of which 1423 individuals had known lifespans to analyse. Amongst these, cause of death was known for 302 individuals.

2.2.3.1 Lifespan and Causes of Death

Analysis of lifespan and causes of death resulted in a mean lifespan of 7.84 ± 2.66 years. Females lived significantly longer than males. Within the population with known causes of death, males were at a significantly increased risk of Dilatative Cardiomyopathy, and females were at a significantly increased risk of cancer other than osteogenic sarcoma. No information on castration status was available.

When comparing dogs born in the 1960s and dogs born after 1980, a highly significant decrease in mean lifespan of about 1½ years was found in the latter population. Significant lifespan differences were also observed in the 1st-generation progeny of 13 popular sires (defined as having more than 10 direct descendants with known lifespan in the data). No significant correlations between lifespan and Wright's Inbreeding Coefficients over 5, 10 and 20 generations as well as Meuwissen's Inbreeding Coefficients were found.

2.2.3.2 Pedigree Analysis

Irish Wolfhounds were found to be extremely inbred, with one ancestor explaining over 25% and three ancestors explaining over 50% of the genetic variability of the population born between 1965 and 2005. While average 10-generation Wright's Inbreeding Coefficients tended to decrease since about 1980, average Meuwissen's Inbreeding Coefficients over the same period remained constant, identifying the above decrease as an artefact caused by the growing population.

Four distinct genetic bottlenecks were identified in the history of the modern Irish Wolfhound population, dating from the 3rd quarter of the 19th century and the times around World War I and II respectively. An exponential increase in the number of dogs born per year could be observed since about 1965

2.2.3.3 Ancestor Analysis of Different Diseases

10-generation ancestor analyses were carried out for individuals affected with Dilatative Cardiomyopathy (DCM), osteogenic sarcoma (OS), gastric dilation and volvulus (GDV), and portosystemic shunt (PSS) and compared to a randomly selected reference population of similar structure regarding countries and years of birth. Ancestor differences between affected and reference populations were found for DCM and OS, but were similar for both diseases. More distinct differences were found in the case of PSS. This condition was further analysed using pedigree diagrams, and possible originators in the ancestor population were identified.

2.3 Discussion and Conclusions (chapter 7)

The third part discusses the findings of the previous chapters, their implications for future breeding strategies, suggestions for further research and also contains a general discussion of the ethics of breeding Irish Wolfhounds.

2.3.1 Lifespan

According to the literature, the early accumulation of oxidative damage during growth plays an important role in the reduced lifespan observed in large and giant dog breeds. Even though there is some disagreement between the different lifespan estimates for Irish Wolfhounds, and despite the right censored data influence this study found, it is abundantly clear that the breed has a generally poor life expectancy, and that steps should be taken to improve the situation. It is possible that Irish Wolfhound life expectancy varies between different countries, although other mechanisms could also have influenced this result.

It is hypothesised that the observed decrease in average lifespan since the 1960s could be caused by a lack of health-related selection pressure due to the increased availability of veterinary care (antibiotics and vaccines) since these times. The exponential increase in numbers since these times may also have contributed to such a decrease in selection pressure, as may the increasing tendency to have many small kennels as opposed to a few large ones.

Based on the findings on castration, it is recommended not to routinely castrate male Irish Wolfhounds due to both its lack of benefit regarding lifespan and its increase of osteosarcoma risk. However, it is likely that castration significantly increases life expectancy in female Irish Wolfhounds.

2.3.2 Population Genetics

Irish Wolfhounds have been subject to at least four important genetic bottlenecks during their modern history, with the most recent occurring in the 1950s. This makes the breed highly inbred, which may explain the lack of influence of inbreeding on lifespan found in this study: Inbreeding and bottlenecks can lead to purging phenomena, through which deleterious alleles can be eliminated from an inbred population.

The high inbreeding level in Irish Wolfhounds today tends to be masked due to the exponential population growth in recent times; in fact, there is an artificial decrease in 10-generation Wright's inbreeding coefficients in more recent times due to this phenomenon.

The observed ancestor differences for the diseases considered were difficult to interpret in the case of DCM, OS and GDV, since they seemed to be similar in all three diseases. In the case of PSS, however, differences were clearer and lead to the construction of a few pedigree diagrams, through which probable originators of the disease could be identified.

Due to the frequent bottlenecks during population history, it was impossible to track any of these diseases further back than the 1950's. Therefore, it cannot be excluded that PSS originated in the ancestors of the probable originators found. However, this consideration is largely irrelevant to present-day breeding practices, given that these pre-bottleneck ancestors are to be found in the pedigrees of all Irish Wolfhounds alive today.

2.3.3 Ethical Considerations

The breeding of Irish Wolfhounds is studied under the premise that ethical questions are raised whenever canine and human interests oppose each other. The ethical implications of both a decreased lifespan and the acceptance of hereditary diseases in breeding practices are discussed, leading to the conclusion that a decrease in lifespan is an ethical problem independent from the occurrence of hereditary diseases. Furthermore, although it is unrealistic to assume that a complete elimination of hereditary disease from the breed will be possible, there are measures that can be expected to result in a significant decrease. The breeders' ethical obligation to put the dogs' interests above their own in these cases is also stressed. A particular and unusual ethical problem is then discussed based on the case study of portosystemic shunt.

2.3.4 Future Prospects in Breeding

Selection against hereditary diseases should be based on their potential impact on the animals' well-being, their frequency throughout the population and the chance of success of appropriate breeding measures. To reach this goal, an open Irish Wolfhound health database would be an extremely useful tool on which to base selection decisions. Given that there are prevalence differences in hereditary diseases amongst different Irish Wolfhound populations, it is impossible to suggest a universally valid breeding strategy for the overall population that incorporates all possible hereditary diseases. However, Dilatative Cardiomyopathy and portosystemic shunt are suggested as prime candidates for selection, considering their global prevalence and high heritability, as well as the availability of diagnostic tests. Based on the breed's genetic history and current population size, it is stated that the potential for severe health- and vigour-based selection was never as good in Irish Wolfhounds as it is today.

2.3.5 Future Research Prospects

Thanks to the ever-increasing communication on the internet, it is possible to locate large pedigree databases of various dog breeds and to obtain copies of some of them for scientific study. There is a large potential for veterinary genetic research analogous to this study in such databases, which has not been realised to-date. The present database and others of its type would also be an interesting base to investigate the heritability of lifespan in the domestic dog, which has not been studied yet.

In Irish Wolfhounds in particular, the oxidative damage model of aging would be interesting to study by establishing the effect of antioxidant substances given during the growth phase on overall life expectancy. As far as inbreeding is concerned, its relation to fertility parameters also suggests itself to be studied, which was done after the first edition of this study. Finally, the present data could also be helpful in the future search for DNA markers associated with certain hereditary diseases, none of which have yet been discovered in Irish Wolfhounds.

Keywords: Irish Wolfhound, dog, population genetics, review, hereditary diseases, lifespan, inbreeding, pedigree analysis, dog breeding, ethics in breeding

3 Literature Review

Several disease predispositions have been reported in Irish Wolfhounds. This section provides a review of the published literature on health conditions and general longevity in the breed and mentions currently ongoing research. While it strives to give as complete as possible a review of the Wolfhound-related material published in the veterinary literature, it does not pretend to be able to cover every disease that occurs in the breed. Irish Wolfhounds are dogs and, as such, can be affected by the complete range of diseases found in this species.

3.1 Lifespan in General

3.1.1 Bias in Lifespan Studies

3.1.1.1 Submitter's Bias

An important consideration in the collection of lifespan and disease data – especially if data collection is performed through questionnaires – is Submitter's Bias: Out of both emotional and economical interests, breeders can be motivated to selectively enter older dogs, which leads to an overestimation of lifespan values. The same mechanisms can also lead to an underestimation regarding the prevalence of certain health conditions. This problem might be less important with private owners, who generally do not have data of many dogs to contribute.

Another variant of Submitter's Bias may occur if data is collected from veterinary medical databases. Complicated cases are usually overrepresented in data from veterinary referral centres, and data from studies of a specific disease is, of course, biased towards the disease in question.

3.1.1.2 Classification Bias

The problem of an accurate diagnosis is another concern in data collection from private individuals. While in the case of Wolfhounds, the diagnoses of Osteosarcoma and Gastric Dilation Volvulus are not difficult to make and a standardised diagnosis of Dilated Cardiomyopathy has become considerably easier through echocardiography and standard diagnostic thresholds (Vollmar 1999 b), unspecific submissions such as "heart disease" still represent a certain classification challenge.

3.1.1.3 Cohort Bias (Right Censored Data)

During analysis of the lifespan studies published in the past, it became clear that many of them were tainted with a phenomenon that can be described as "Cohort Bias": A misleading decrease of the measured lifespan when dogs are sorted by year of death rather than year of birth, which is due to right censored data (Kalbfleisch and Prentice 1980).

The nature of this bias is not apparent when considering the time of death; however, it becomes obvious when considering the time of birth: In order for a set of lifespan data to be representative, all dogs born during the considered time span must already be dead. If this is not the case, the average lifespan will seemingly (and falsely) drop. The extent of this bias depends on the structure of the available longevity data – in Wolfhounds, dogs born less than 12 years before the end of the data collection period can be expected to be subject to it. Naturally, the bias grows stronger as the whelping date approaches the end of the data collection period (Urfer 2008).

In explaining this to a lay public, the author has found the following example to be very useful: If we imagine a litter of 10 individuals born 6 years ago, out of which 3 dogs died at age 5, this does not imply that the average lifespan for the litter was five years. Average lifespan can only be determined after all 10 dogs are dead. This is obvious when we consider the year of birth, but becomes masked when considering the year of death.

3.1.2 Scientific Publications

3.1.2.1 Comfort

While it is generally agreed upon that Wolfhounds as a breed have a below-average life expectancy, relatively little scientific work has been done on the topic. The first paper on the subject was published 50 years ago based on individuals born in one kennel between 1927 and 1945 (Comfort 1956). It found a median age at death of 4.95 ± 0.94 years for males and 6.59 ± 0.95 years for females who had survived their first year of life. The maximum ages in his sample of 154 animals were 10.5 years in males and 13.42 years in females.

Comfort found a high mortality during the first year of life, with a chance of reaching one year of age of only 61.29% for males and 72.92% for females born alive. Interestingly, the overall survival curve was linear rather than sigmoid, indicating a relatively high mortality at a young age. Given that effective vaccines and antibiotics were not available at the time, this high death rate was probably caused by infectious diseases.

Although Comfort does not give the relative importance of different causes of death for the overall population, he mentions that of the twelve males who died in their third year of life, four died from distemper, four from gastroenteritis, two of infectious pneumonia, one of unknown causes and one was "destroyed as a result of persistent fits".

In the older animals, Comfort found that three of the four oldest males died of "heart disease", while the three oldest bitches all died of mammary carcinoma. One nine-year-old bitch died of uterine carcinoma, and no tumours were recorded in any of the males. This is a remarkable observation when considering the high incidence of Osteogenic sarcoma in the breed nowadays (see chapter 3.4).

While he did not investigate the relation between lifespan and inbreeding, Comfort argued that Wolfhounds had probably reached a point where a stable lifespan was established that would not be subject to further inbreeding depression, comparable to the situation that occurs in inbred strains of *Drosophila melanogaster*.

In a follow-up study, Comfort provided survival information of an additional ten Wolfhounds from the same kennel, which were not significantly different from his previous results (Comfort 1960). No information as to their whelping dates or causes of death was provided.

The Comfort studies are certainly a very valuable 'glimpse of the past'. However, it must also be noted that their focus on one family of dogs from one single kennel is somewhat problematic if we want to extrapolate Comfort's findings on the whole Wolfhound population of the time. Unfortunately, the degree of a possible Cohort Bias (if any) cannot be deduced from his published data either.

3.1.2.2 Deeb and Wolf

Deeb and Wolf (1994) evaluated data from the Veterinary Medical Database of Purdue University (www.vmdb.org) of dogs that had died between Jan. 1, 1982 and Sept. 30, 1992. This included n=116 Irish Wolfhounds. 30 % of these died before age 4, 40 % between ages 4 and 7, 25% between ages 7 and 10, and 5% lived to over 10 years of age (Deeb and Wolf 1994).

The period of death data collection and its grouping by year of death makes it clear that these results are tainted with Cohort Bias.

3.1.2.3 Li, Deeb et al.

Li, Deeb et al. (1996) published an article on in vitro proliferative capacity of dermal fibroblasts as a function of body size in dogs and showed that while there were no gender differences, Wolfhound (and Great Dane) fibroblasts had a significantly lower proliferative capacity than fibroblasts taken from dogs of other breeds in the same age class. However, no such correlation was found in other large (but not giant) breeds.

The paper included a lifespan evaluation of n=236 Wolfhounds provided by the Veterinary Medical Database of Purdue University (www.vmdb.org), which found that 62% died between 4 to 7 years of age, 32% died between 7 and 10 years, and 6% died between 10 and 15 years. No reference as to causes of death and/or their percentual importance was given (Li, Deeb et al. 1996).

The death class of dogs between 10 and 15 years was arbitrarily set by the Purdue Veterinary Medical Database and might be misleading in the sense that, considering the rest of the available data as well as the findings of the study at hand, it is highly improbable that a significant number of Wolfhounds lived past 12 years of age in this dataset. Furthermore, it is probable that the data used were also right censored, although the extent to which this was the case remains unknown due to the fact that no information on death years is given. Similarly, the lack of a death group before age 4 implies the presence of left censored data, which also reduces the significance of these findings as far as lifespan is concerned.

3.1.2.4 Michell

Michell (1999) conducted a survey of British dog owners concerning cause of and age at death of the last dog these owners had had. Nine Irish Wolfhounds were included in the answers. Mean age was 6.2 years; inter-quartile range was 4.8 years. 8 (89%) of these dogs had died from unspecified cancers (Michell 1999). The study was tainted with Cohort Bias.

3.1.2.5 Egenvall, Bonnett et al.

Egenvall, Bonnett et al. (2005) published estimated survival curves calculated from data of dogs registered by a Swedish pet insurance company between 1995 and 2000, including a population of 1957 Irish Wolfhound dog years at risk (DYAR). The analysis was limited to individuals up to 10 years of age and included probabilities of death by ages 5, 8 and 10 as well as survival chances dependent on age. The results are given in table 3.1.

Probability of death by:			Given survival to 5, chance of death by 8	Given survival to 8, chance of death by 10
5 years	8 years	10 years		
28 %	63 %	91 %	49 %	76 %

Table 3.1: Survival chances of insured Irish Wolfhounds in Sweden that died between 1995 and 2000 (Egenvall, Bonnett et al. 2005).

The death cohorts used in the study make it clear that these data are right censored.

3.1.3 Lay Publications

3.1.3.1 Bernardi

27 years after Comfort's second paper, Bernardi published the results of an anonymised retrospective owner survey on lifespan and causes of death in Irish Wolfhounds in the United States between 1966 and 1986 (Bernardi 1986). She found a mean age at death of 6.47 years in her population of 582 dogs (291 males, 274 females, 17 unspecified). Ages in males ranged from 0.5 to 13.5 years, with a mean of 6 years, whereas ages in females ranged from 0.58 to 12.53 years, with a mean age of 6.55 years.

As opposed to Comfort, Bernardi also analysed the percentual importance of different causes of death, which will be quoted in the following chapters focusing on causes of death. Unfortunately, her study did not include any significance analyses, which are therefore delivered in chapter 5.1.

In an addendum to her study, Bernardi observes that the average lifespan did not increase when she removed deaths by cancer, Cardiovascular disease and Gastric Dilation Volvulus and suggests that these figures would seem to dispel any hope that longevity could be improved by eliminating a certain disease and that the problem therefore is more complex than mere susceptibility to specific diseases. However, this statement ignores the probable outcome that the dogs affected with the excluded diseases would probably have lived longer if they had not died from said diseases. It may also reflect the existence other mechanisms contributing to longevity (see chapter 7.1.1).

Further analysis of Bernardi's original data performed during the study at hand showed that her findings are subject to Cohort Bias. When this bias was excluded, the average ages were significantly higher than what she had found (see chapter 5.1.1).

3.1.3.2 Murphy

In 1991, Murphy published a pedigree book, which additionally contains lifespan information of 591 individuals born between 1950 and 1990 that she had collected from various breeders in Ireland and the UK (Murphy 1991), but gives no information on the causes of death apart from a few descriptions of a death as accidental. These data were also analysed during the study at hand and Cohort Bias corrected (see chapter 5.1.2).

Murphy also performed an analysis of her data sorted by kennel names, where she investigated how many individuals from different kennels had lived past 8 years of age (Murphy 1996). Unfortunately, this list was not adjusted for the total number of individuals produced by the kennels in question, which makes it impossible to compare the percentual chance of these kennels to produce Wolfhounds that live beyond 8 in any meaningful way.

3.1.3.3 Prokopenko

The most recent attempt to investigate lifespan and causes of death in Wolfhounds was conducted in the form of an online survey containing 139 individuals of which the results were published online (Prokopenko 1998). It found an average life expectancy of 6.41 years, but was also subject to Cohort Bias. When this bias was corrected, the average life expectancy increased similarly to Bernardi's original data (see chapter 5.1.1).

Much like Bernardi, Prokopenko also investigated the percentual importance of different causes of death. Her findings will be quoted in the following chapters.

3.1.3.4 Miscellaneous

Starbuck and Howell briefly touch the subject in writing that "many people ask about Wolfhound longevity. Wolfhounds are much the same as other large breeds, though not so full of years as some smaller breeds such as Terriers. We have sold many that lived from eleven to fourteen years, and a few that lived longer, but they are the exception" (p. 151) (Starbuck and Howell 1969).

Donnelly states that stress is an important contributor to a shortened lifespan in Wolfhounds and recommends to reduce it as much as possible. In an addendum, it is mentioned that "Mr. Donnelly has six Irish Wolfhounds at present, two aged 14 years, one 10 years, one 9 years and the two 'pups' at four years. The oldest hound he had was 15 years" (Donnelly 1976).

Hudson states that "the Irish Wolfhound in its native climate, i.e. the British Isles, generally reaches from eight to ten years though some blood strains only just make seven. Abroad and especially in dry hot climates they do not seem to last so long and have about six years of active life" (p. 51). No source is given (Hudson 1981).

Heffels writes that "due to the size of the breed, Wolfhounds unfortunately only live to 9 to 12 years, provided that they are kept and cared for in an optimal way." (vol. I, p. 56). No source is given (Heffels 1989).

McBryde mentions that "the average age reached by a male Wolfhound in Britain is about 6.5 years; in the USA, it is only 5.5 years. Females live on average a year or so longer. However, these are average life-spans and do include puppy deaths as well as hounds with much longer life-spans of up to 13 years" (p. 85). No source is given (McBryde 1998).

On the other hand, Gover writes that "nowadays, nine is considered a very good age for a hound, ten years and over being exceptional, and with present-day health-related problems (...), the expected lifespan is currently about 7.5 years. Some bloodlines seem to live longer than others, but no difference has been shown between dogs and bitches" (p. 103). No source is given (Gover 1998).

Most recently, Kane writes that "while some bloodlines seem to live longer than others, the expected lifespan is about seven to eight years, with nine or ten considered a very long life" (p. 38). No source is given (Kane 2001).

Furthermore, many Wolfhound clubs periodically publish a "list of veterans". Since such data are highly biased towards older animals by their very nature, none of them were included in the present study. Speaking of their general value for breeders, it is of paramount importance that they are set in relation to the number of dogs with a similar genetic makeup for an objective evaluation to be possible.

Currently, a Dutch foundation is maintaining a Wolfhound health and lifespan database on the internet at http://www.iw-database.com/search.php. While it does not contain a large number of dogs at the moment, the concept does have some merit. Concerns regarding Submitter's and Classification Bias apply as specified above.

3.2 Intrahepatic Portosystemic Shunt (PSS)

3.2.1 Description

Portosystemic Shunt in Wolfhounds is a congenital malformation of the porto-caval blood vessels, leading to gastro-intestinal and neurological symptoms. The condition is hereditary (see 3.2.3), but the exact mechanism that causes the Ductus venosus to remain open is not known (Meyer, Rothuizen et al. 1995; White, Burton et al. 1998; Ubbink, van de Broek et al. 1998 b; Hunt 2004).

3.2.1.1 Pathophysiology

In healthy dogs, blood rich in nutriments and ammonia coming from the intestine is transported through the portal vein to the liver, where it passes through a capillary system and its many components are chemically modified and detoxified before being released into the main circulatory system. In the foetus, this mechanism is not necessary, and the capillary system of the liver is therefore bypassed by the Ductus venosus, which closes soon after birth in healthy dogs (Broome, Walsh et al. 2004).

In Irish Wolfhounds affected with PSS, this vessel fails to occlude after birth, which causes a leaking of toxic metabolic products into the bloodstream, leading to the typical symptoms of hepatic encephalopathy. Anatomically, the persistent Ductus venosus is located intrahepatically, most commonly in the left liver division (White, Burton et al. 1998).

3.2.1.2 Symptoms

Patients with PSS often exhibit non-specific symptoms such as stunted growth, intermittent anorexia, depression, vomiting, PU/PD and behavioural changes. Signs of hepatic encephalopathy (ataxia, stupor, head pressing, seizures etc.) are often intermittent and usually worsen after feeding, especially when a high protein diet is used (Watson and Herrtage 1998; Fossum and Hedlund 2002). Affected dogs typically develop symptoms before one year of age (Broome, Walsh et al. 2004).

3.2.1.3 Diagnosis

Most affected animals are microhepatic on X-rays (Fossum and Hedlund 2002), and it is usually possible to demonstrate an intrahepatic PSS through ultrasonography (Suter and Niemand 2001 a). Scintigraphy following rectal administration of TcO_4 is another possible way of diagnosis: If a shunt is present, the marker reaches the heart before or at the same time it reaches the liver (Bernhardt, Westhoff et al. 1996).

Haematological signs may include normochromic microcytosis, mild nonregenerative anaemia, target cell formation or poikilocytosis. Plasma albumin and BUN may be lowered due to reduced liver function. ALAT, ASAT and AP may be slightly raised, while serum bilirubin is usually normal (Fossum and Hedlund 2002). Urate crystals may be found in the urine of up to 50% of affected dogs (Suter and Niemand 2001 a).

Wolfhound puppies can be screened for the presence of a PSS from about six weeks of age by measuring postprandial serum bile acid levels between 90 and 120 minutes after feeding. A deliberately low threshold value of 30 µmol per litre is set in order to reach high sensitivity, and individuals that have higher scores should be subjected to a dynamic bile acid test (comparison of pre- and postprandial bile acid levels). If the dynamic test result remains positive, more invasive diagnostic measures are indicated (Kerr and van Doorn 1999).

Another common test for PSS in dogs is the measuring of plasma ammonia levels. However, it must be noted in this context that physiological fasting ammonia levels are higher in young Wolfhounds than they are in other breeds and that fasting ammonia levels below 120 µmol per litre should therefore not be considered indicative of a PSS. There is an overlap between healthy and affected individuals at ammonia levels between 120 and 125 µmol per litre, however (Meyer, Rothuizen et al. 1996).

Other results show even more of an overlap of ammonia levels in Wolfhounds, with affected individuals tested at values as low as 121 µmol per litre and healthy individuals tested at values as high as 127 µmol per litre. Furthermore, it is necessary to measure plasma ammonia immediately after the blood sample is taken due to its volatile nature, while bile acid levels are stable enough for serum samples to be sent to a laboratory, making the bile acid test a more practical tool for clinical mass screening (Kerr 1996).

On a related note, it has recently been shown that both sensitivity and specificity of a fasting bile acid test are considerably lower than those of serum ammonia testing. However, Irish Wolfhounds were excluded from this study due to their breed-specific juvenile metabolic hyperammonaemia mentioned above (Gerritzen-Bruning, van den Ingh et al. 2006).

In suspected individuals, ammonia tolerance testing is another possibility: Plasma ammonia is measured in the fasting animal. Subsequently, 100 mg/kg of ammonium chloride is entered into the stomach through a gastric probe and plasma ammonia measured again after 30 minutes. Levels significantly higher than 120 µmol per litre are considered a positive result (Kraft 2000).

It has been shown that the aforementioned increased ammonia levels in healthy juvenile Wolfhounds are not caused by a delayed closure of the Ductus venosus and thus seem to be a metabolic idiosyncrasy of the breed. Plasma ammonia levels were shown to have decreased markedly by 13 weeks of age and are normal in adult Wolfhounds, indicating the existence of a spontaneous remission process (Meyer, Rothuizen et al. 1996). Biochemically, the transient increase in ammonia levels seems to be caused by enzyme deficiencies in the urea cycle, which can gradually be compensated through alternative metabolic pathways as the dogs mature (Zandvliet and Rothuizen 2007).

3.2.1.4 Therapy and Prognosis

While it is possible to manage PSS conservatively through a low-protein diet, lactulose and antibiotic treatment, survival time of such animals is reduced markedly, more so in intrahepatic than in extrahepatic shunts. While there seems to be an improvement in gastrointestinal symptoms, a worsening tendency could be observed in the case of neurological symptoms (Watson and Herrtage 1998).

Conservative therapy is also indicated to stabilise animals that exhibit signs of hepatic encephalopathy before surgery is attempted and should additionally include fluid therapy and the normalisation of acid-base disturbances. Antibiotic treatment (neomycin, metronidazole, ampicillin) is also indicated to reduce the production of bacterial toxins in the intestine (Fossum and Hedlund 2002).

Surgery is the therapy of choice, but complication and mortality rates are high. The technique of choice is reported to be direct posthepatic ligation of the shunt vessel (White, Burton et al. 1998). Another reported technique is cellophane banding, which was used in two Wolfhound puppies, one of which survived (Connery, McAllister et al. 2002). For intrahepatic PSS, postoperative complications have been reported in 77% of cases, short-term mortality is reported to range from 11% to 28% and overall mortality from 23% to 63.6%. The one-year survival rate was reported as 61%, while the two-year survival rate was 55% (Papazoglou, Monnet et al. 2002). Claims of lower complication rates that are occasionally made by breeders are not supported by the available evidence.

Recently, there have been reports of successful shunt attenuations through minimally invasive coil embolisation and other occlusion techniques using a jugular venous approach (Leveille, Johnson et al. 2003; Weisse, Mondschein et al. 2005). While results seem to be promising to-date, these techniques should still be considered experimental at the moment given the small number of described cases.

3.2.2 Epizootology

According to the veterinary literature, PSS incidence rates in the Irish Wolfhound population are reported to vary between 2.1 and 3.4% of all puppies and 18% of all litters. Smaller litters seem to have a higher risk (Meyer, Rothuizen et al. 1995; Ubbink, van de Broek et al. 1998 b; Kerr and van Doorn 1999). As is the case with surgery complication rates, lay claims of lower incidence rates are not supported by the available evidence. According to Hardy-Weinberg ($p^2+2pq+q^2=1$; $p+q=1$), the published numbers imply a healthy carrier frequency of 24.8% to 30.1% of all Irish Wolfhounds (also see 3.2.3 below).

Furthermore, PSS incidence rates in the direct descendants of certain individuals have been measured to be as high as 15% (Ubbink, van de Broek et al. 1998 a).

3.2.3 Heredity and Control Measures

Intrahepatic PSS has been described to be passed on in a simple autosomal recessive way (Rothuizen 2002). More recently, the same research group has published evidence that is not compatible with such a mode of inheritance and proposes that PSS in the breed can be explained by a digenic, triallelic mode of inheritance (van Steenbeek, Leegwater et al. 2009). This would imply the existence of a major PSS locus in combination with a separate modifier locus, which would interact epistaticly with the major locus. This mode of inheritance is shown in more detail in table 3.2 below. A genogram of the test matings falsifying the simple autosomal recessive mode of inheritance is provided in figure 3.1.

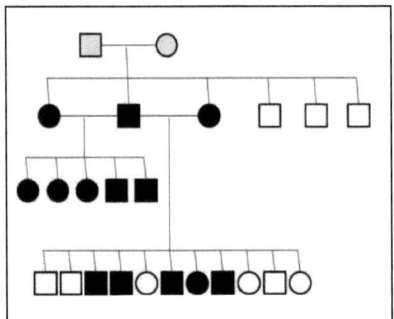

Figure 3.1: Test mating genogram of an affected male and two affected female siblings (van Steenbeek, Leegwater et al. 2009), demonstrating the high heritability, but falsifying the simple autosomal recessive mode of inheritance.

While there is ongoing research on the topic, no marker or gene test that would allow recognising carriers that have not yet produced affected offspring has been made available as of today. While the nature of the data used in the study at hand made it impossible to determine a mode of inheritance, the hereditary nature of PSS could also be demonstrated (see Chapter 7.2.4.2).

Shunt Genotype	Modifier Genotype	Affected?	Shunt Carrier?
PP	00	no	no
PP	10	no	no
PP	11	no	no
Pp	00	no	yes
Pp	10	no	yes
Pp	11	no	yes
pp	00	no	yes
pp	10	yes	yes
pp	11	yes	yes

Table 3.2: Possible digenic, triallelic PSS inheritance in Irish Wolfhounds and its effects on phenotype.

The first published recommendation was not to breed close relatives of affected puppies (Skancke 1994). Later, it was shown that the Dutch breeders had not realised the full potential to select against PSS and that the incidence of the disease was increasing (Meyer, Rothuizen et al. 1995). Risk estimation through cluster analysis of genetic heterogeneity was proposed as a means of selection that did not require the mode of inheritance to be known (Ubbink, van de Broek et al. 1998 b).

Some national breed clubs now require that all puppies be tested for the condition before sale, while others at least encourage breeders to test. However, given that an inherited condition that kills before sexual maturity cannot be passed on through affected individuals, it is logical that identification and elimination of these individuals from the gene pool will not affect incidence and prevalence of the disease. Therefore, testing to identify affected individuals in a litter cannot be expected to reduce the incidence of the disease if the healthy carriers thus identified are not excluded from breeding. To the author's knowledge, the Irish Wolfhound Club of Switzerland is the only breed organisation to exclude parents (certain carriers) and full siblings (2/3 risk of being carriers) of affected Wolfhounds from breeding so far (Anonymous 2002).

Nowadays, the bile acid test as described by Kerr and van Doorn (1999) is widely used to screen Wolfhound puppies for the presence of a PSS, and it has been added to the code of ethics of several clubs that all puppies should be screened before sale. However, the exclusion of carriers from breeding is not commonly requested, which shows that such a screening test has the potential to be abused to primarily serve both the breeders' and buyers' interests instead of the dogs' if it can prevent breeders from selling affected dogs (also see chapter 7.3.3.1).

3.3 Dilatative Cardiomyopathy (DCM)

3.3.1 Description

Dilatative Cardiomyopathy is a primary disease of the heart muscle not usually associated with coronary artery disease and only secondarily affecting heart valve mechanism (Bishop 1986). The disease is hereditary in Irish Wolfhounds (see 3.3.3): Several mechanisms and candidate loci have been and are still being discussed, yet the underlying molecular mechanisms remain unknown (Broschk 2004).

3.3.1.1 Pathophysiology

The disease is characterised by a marked loss of myocardial contractility, leading to impaired systolic ventricular function and also impairing diastolic function. These impairments result in elevated ventricular end-diastolic atrial and venous pressures and ultimately in congestive heart failure. The reduction in ventricular stroke volume leads to systemic arterial hypotension. Due to the dilation of the heart muscle, functional insufficiency of both the tricuspid and the mitral valve is usually present in the later stages of the disease, but the degree of regurgitation is usually mild (Vollmar 1998; Fox, Sisson et al. 1999).

Ultrastructurally, one study of large breed DCM found intermyofibrillar spaces, myofibrillar degeneration, lipofuscin granules, fat droplets, myelin figures, mitochondrial hyperplasia, disruption of myofibrils and Z band thickening. All of these features (except Z band thickening) can also be found in the heart muscle of clinically healthy dogs, although to a much smaller degree. Mitochondrial hyperplasia and disruption of myofibrils were described as having a similar extent in 46 sections from eight DCM cases in giant dogs. These findings are not specific for DCM, however, but rather reflect long standing ventricular hypertrophy with subsequent congestive heart failure (Bishop 1986).

A more recent study found that giant breed DCM is characterised by thin attenuated wavy myocardial fibres as opposed to the "fatty infiltration degenerative" type seen in Doberman Pinschers and Boxers (Tidholm and Jonsson 2005).

Additionally, some animals seem to exhibit high-grade panarteriitis of the larger cardiac arteries, especially in the left ventricular wall and the interventricular septum, leading to particular obstruction of the lumen (Broschk 2004).

3.3.1.2 Symptoms

In Wolfhounds, DCM goes through a long subclinical stage that is mainly characterised by atrial fibrillation (AF) as mentioned above. Contrary to "lone atrial fibrillation" in humans, this seems to be an objective risk factor for the eventual development of DCM to the point that it can be said that Wolfhounds with AF can be considered to likely be in a stage of "occult DCM" (Koch, Pedersen et al. 1996; Vollmar 1996; Brownlie and Cobb 1999).

Weight loss, combined with extreme tachycardia, dyspnoea and ascites are reported to be the typical symptoms of clinically manifest Wolfhound DCM. These and other signs of progressive cardiac failure, such as exercise intolerance, coughing and general apathy are usually indicative of an advanced stage of the disease (Brownlie and Cobb 1999).

3.3.1.3 Diagnosis

Echocardiography is the gold standard for the diagnosis of canine DCM (Fox, Sisson et al. 1999). Reference values for healthy Wolfhounds and exact values for diagnostic parameters were published in 1999 (Vollmar 1999 a; Vollmar 1999 b). Parameters with highly significant variability between the groups of normal dogs, subclinically affected dogs (occult DCM) and clinically affected dogs are given in table 3.3. In this context, it is interesting to note that Brownlie and Cobb (1999) do not consider fractional shortening a reliable indicator of the presence of DCM in Irish Wolfhounds.

Measurement	Normal ± SD	P1	Occult ± SD	P2	Advanced ± SD
LVIDs (mm)	35.4 (2.8)	<0.001	42.1 (4.4)	<0.001	52.4 (8.0)
LVIDd (mm)	53.2 (4.0)	<0.001	60.1 (6.4)	0.00027	67.4 (6.2)
FS (%)	34.0 (4.5)	<0.001	25.6 (4.5)	0.020	20.7 (8.3)
LA (mm) M-Mode	32.9 (3.4)	<0.001	42.4 (9.2)	NS	47.3 (11.1)
EPSS (mm)	6.8 (1.6)	<0.001	10.3 (1.0)	0.028	13.4 (5.2)
LA (mm) 2D	47.3 (4.3)	<0.001	54.9 (5.5)	0.0067	71.2 (18.6)
ESVI (ml/m^2)	28.7 (5.7)	<0.001	56.9 (8.1)	0.0049	105.7 (59.2)

Table 3.3: Mean measurements ± Standard Deviation of echocardiographic parameters with highly significant differences between groups. Taken from (Vollmar 1999 b). P1 = difference between normal dogs and dogs with occult DCM (unpaired 2-tailed Student's t-test); P2 = difference between dogs with occult DCM and dogs with clinical signs of DCM (unpaired 2-tailed Student's t-test). NS=not significant; LVIDs and LVIDd = end-systolic and end-diastolic left ventricular internal dimensions; FS = fractional shortening; LA (M-Mode) = left atrial diameter during systole by M-mode; EPSS = E-point to septal separation; LA 2D = systolic left atrial diameter; ESVI = end-systolic volume index.

While fully developed clinical DCM is comparably easy to diagnose, it is important for optimal treatment to catch the disease in an early stage. On auscultation, low-pitched protodiastolic gallop sounds are indicative of DCM, as are pulse deficits, absolute arrhythmia and tachyarrhythmia. In about half of the dogs with DCM, a soft regurgitant systolic murmur can also be heard (Fox, Sisson et al. 1999).

Electrocardiographically, AF is the most consistent ECG sign found in Wolfhounds with DCM. Other abnormities may include ventricular and supraventricular premature contractions (VPC's and SVPC's), P mitrale and 1st and 2nd degree AV-block. Bigeminal rhythm and paroxysmal tachycardia can also be observed. It is also possible for a Wolfhound with DCM to have an entirely normal ECG, although this must be considered rare (Brownlie 1991; Harpster 1994; Brownlie and Cobb 1999; Vollmar 2000).

3.3.1.4 Therapy

The ultimate treatment goal would be to reverse the underlying disease process responsible for DCM before irreversible damage to the myocardium has occurred. Since the underlying mechanism is unknown in Wolfhounds, the goals must be pragmatically reduced to identifying and reversing any underlying cause of heart failure, to reduce the clinical symptoms, to improve the quality of life and to decrease mortality. The exact treatment must be tailored to the individual patient.

Patients presenting with signs of acute heart failure should be treated with an i.v. combination of furosemide and sodium nitroprusside, the latter being a potent, ultra-short acting vasodilator that must be infused continually to remain effective. Additionally, the β_1-agonist dobutamine can be infused, although it must not be mixed with sodium nitroprusside. Most dogs can be switched from i.v. to oral administration of drugs within 48 hours (Fox, Sisson et al. 1999).

DCM is incurable at present, making treatment lifelong. Its cornerstone at present is the inhibition of angiotensin converting enzyme through an ACE-inhibitor (enalapril, benazepril etc). Enalapril maleate has been shown to significantly increase survival time in canine DCM (Ettinger, Benitz et al. 1998).

Since AF by itself reduces cardiac output by about 25%, it should also be addressed in the treatment. Digoxin is indicated to reduce AF and tachycardia and can be combined with β-adrenergic receptor blockers or calcium channel blockers, the latter being reported as the most effective drug to reduce heart rate, although in long-term treatment, β-blockers may have more beneficial effects on myocardial function. Since there are marked individual differences in sensitivity to this class of drugs, the initial dose should be low and then be raised gradually until the desired effect is achieved. The effect on overall survival has not been studied in dogs (Fox, Sisson et al. 1999).

On a side note, the author is aware of several cases where electrical atrial defibrillation was attempted in Wolfhounds with varying success. The technique has also been described in the literature (Osswald, Trouton et al. 1998).

Solatol and other class III antiarrhythmic drugs are an additional possibility for the treatment of ventricular arrhythmias in canine DCM, but there are no studies on its effectivity in dogs as of now. However, there is anecdotal evidence of its benefits where other antiarrhythmic drugs had failed (Fox, Sisson et al. 1999).

A relatively recent development is the addition of the calcium-sensitising inodilator pimobendan to standard treatment with furosemide, enalapril and digoxin, which was shown to increase survival in Doberman Pinschers, but not in English Cocker Spaniels (Fuentes, Corcoran et al. 2002). Pimobendan was also reported to increase survival in a hamster model of hereditary Cardiomyopathy (van Meel, Mauz et al. 1989). However, some results from human medicine suggest that there may be an increased mortality in the long term (Mathew and Katz 1998; Fox, Sisson et al. 1999).

While thrombosis is not a usual complication of DCM in dogs, left atrial thrombi have been identified at autopsy in Wolfhounds with DCM, and it might therefore be indicated to add anticoagulants (e.g. aspirin or warfarin) to the treatment regimen (Brownlie and Cobb 1999).

Surgical treatment techniques have also been described. While in humans, the treatment of choice is a heart transplant, such operations are not usually performed in dogs. Successful dynamic cardiomyoplasty, the covering of both ventricles with an envelope of skeletal muscle (usually the right M. latissimus dorsi) which is then connected to a pacemaker, has been used in humans since 1985 and is also described as a clinical therapy for canine DCM (Aklog, Murphy et al. 1994; Monnet and Orton 1994; Orton, Monnet et al. 1994). Prosthetic cardiac binding and adynamic (no pacemaking of the muscle graft) cardiomyoplasty have also shown a positive effect in the treatment of experimentally induced canine DCM (Oh, Badhwar et al. 1998). However, these techniques are not currently in wide clinical use.

Cellular cardiomyoplasty is another experimental technique that involves the injection of previously cultured autologous skeletal muscle cells into the heart muscle. While there have been promising results so far in hamsters, only very limited data are available for dogs with DCM (Borenstein, Chetboul et al. 2002).

3.3.1.5 Prognosis

Survival time is highly variable from one individual to the next, which makes it basically impossible to predict how long a dog is going to survive on treatment. At least in cases presenting with advanced heart failure, it is recommended to observe the animal's individual reaction to therapy before making a tentative prognosis based on these observations (Fox, Sisson et al. 1999). An early initiation of treatment with ACE inhibitors and (where indicated) digoxin or antiarrhythmic drugs seems to influence the course of the disease in a positive way (Vollmar 2000).

One study recorded survival times in a population of 98 Wolfhounds with DCM without standardised treatment and found an average survival of 5.1 months in the 39 dogs that died as a result of DCM, while it was 15.7 months in the dogs that were still alive when the study was completed. The exact results are given in table 3.4.

It is worth noting that survival time in Irish Wolfhounds affected with DCM is usually longer than in other breeds where it has been studied. This can be explained by three factors: First, pleural effusion rather than pulmonary oedema is the prevailing symptom in Wolfhound CHF, which can develop over several weeks before more severe clinical signs are observed. Second, left ventricular function does not become as severely impaired as in other breeds with DCM and usually reacts well to positive inotropic therapy. Third, extreme tachycardia is induced by AF, which often reacts favourably to digoxin and other antiarrhythmic drugs, reducing further deterioration that is normally induced by tachycardia (Vollmar 2000).

Parameters	n	Median (mos)	Range (mos)
Mild to moderate CHF, still alive	26	14	2.0 - 33
Mild to moderate CHF, dead	18	5.5	0.07 - 35
Advanced CHF, dead	17	2.75	0.2 - 14
Occult DCM, still alive	33	17	0.25 - 68
Occult DCM, dead	4	13	10 - 28

Table 3.4: Survival times of 98 Irish Wolfhounds diagnosed with DCM; taken from Vollmar (2000). Treatment not standardised. CHF = Congestive Heart Failure

One study suggests that AF in combination with multifocal ventricular dysrhythmia is a negative prognostic sign for Wolfhounds with DCM (Brownlie and Cobb 1999), while another study found a correlation between the prevalence of supraventricular cardiac arrhythmias (mainly AF) and girth in male Wolfhounds and a similar correlation with both height at shoulder and girth in female Wolfhounds. However, the authors add that this does not necessarily imply a cause-effect relation, as these variables may be dependent on a third, unknown factor (Brownlie and Nott 1991).

3.3.2 Epizootology

Numbers published in studies on the prevalence of DCM in the breed differ somewhat. An overview is given in table 3.5.

Authors	n	prev. DCM (%)	prev. AF (%)	Country
(Bohn, Patterson et al. 1971)	24	N/A	4.16	USA
(Bernardi 1986)	582	15.1*	N/A	USA
(Brownlie 1991)	496	N/A	10.5	UK
(Vollmar 1996)	170	14.1	16.5	Germany
(Prokopenko 1998)	139	14.4*	N/A	USA/CDN
(Vollmar 1998)	393	16.3	13.4	Ger/NL
(Brownlie and Cobb 1999)	995	3.9**	11.6	UK
(Vollmar 1999 b)	400	16.5	N/A	Germany
(Vollmar 2000)	500	24.2	23.4	Germany
(Vollmar and Fox 2001)	232	12.1	16.4	NW Europe
(Broschk 2004)	997	27.1***	N/A	Ger/NL/B
(Egenvall, Bonnett et al. 2006)	85	44.7****	N/A	Sweden
Urfer (2007) – present study	468	20.51*	N/A	Worldwide
Urfer (2007) – Cohort Bias removed	302	18.54*	N/A	Worldwide

Table 3.5: Prevalence of DCM and AF in Irish Wolfhounds as published in different research studies. *Mortality rates, including cases submitted as 'heart disease'. **May be influenced by loss to follow-up. ***Includes some dogs from Vollmar (2000). ****Mortality rate; dogs over 10 years of age excluded. See chapter 6.2.1.2 for a discussion of the influence of removing Cohort Bias in the present study.

Since the term "Dilatative Cardiomyopathy" (DCM) was not widely used before 1980, it is unclear what the exact diagnosis was in some of the earlier causes. Both Bernardi (1986) and Prokopenko (1998) thus did not use DCM as a death category and stayed with "Cardiovascular disease". The same reservation applies to the older datasets in the study at hand.

While there is no general agreement on whether a sex predisposition exists, males were found to be at an increased risk in the studies where such a predisposition was described (Bernardi 1986; Vollmar 1998; Vollmar 1999 b; Vollmar 2000; Broschk 2004; Egenvall, Bonnett et al. 2006). The results of the present study also support the hypothesis of an increased risk for males (see chapter 6.1.6.2).

3.3.3 Heredity and Control Measures

The assumption that AF may have a hereditary component in Irish Wolfhounds was first brought up in 1994 (Harpster 1994), and further evidence for a familial predisposition was discussed by Vollmar (1996), Brownlie and Cobb (1999), and Vollmar (1999 b).

A familiar pattern of DCM has been observed in Wolfhounds, and it was suggested that an autosomal dominant pattern of inheritance would be fitting to explain the distribution (Cobb, Brownlie et al. 1996; Vollmar 2000). An association of DCM with an increased inbreeding coefficient was also reported (Broschk 2004), which could not be reproduced in the present study relying on more exhaustive pedigree information (see chapter 6.2.3.2)

Complex segregation analysis in a population of 272 Irish Wolfhounds with DCM, taken from 878 screened individuals and combined with pedigree information of a total of 2203 individuals showed that a mixed monogenic-polygenic major gene inheritance model combined with sex-linked expression of the major gene effect best explained the observed DCM. Estimations of the heritability of DCM found in this study ranged from $h^2_{liab} = 38.9 \pm 9.1\%$ to $h^2_{liab} = 50.0 \pm 8.9\%$ using Restricted Maximum Likelihood Estimation and from $h^2 = 58.1 \pm 11.6\%$ to $h^2 = 64.0 \pm 10.2\%$ using the Gibbs Sampling method. A simple monogenic mode of inheritance could be excluded (Broschk 2004; Distl, Vollmar et al. 2007).

Several possible candidate genes for the disease have been studied in the breed, although none of those studied so far have shown any correlation between their occurrence and the occurrence of DCM in Irish Wolfhounds. The candidate genes that have thus been excluded so far are tafazzin (Philipp, Broschk et al. 2007), titin-cap (Philipp, Vollmar et al. 2008 a), cardiac muscle actin alpha, cysteine and glycine-rich protein 3, desmin, phospholamban, sarcoglycan delta and tropomodulin 1 (Philipp, Vollmar et al. 2008 b).

One suggested way of breeding to reduce DCM incidence is to omit using young males and animals with manifest AF (Brownlie and Cobb 1999). Regular standardised heart examination including echocardiography is recommended in all breeding stock (Vollmar 1999 b; Vollmar 2000). Proven healthy parents and grandparents at over 8 years of age provide the most valuable information to determine the risk of developing DCM. It is suggested that the number of litters per dog is to be kept to a maximum of 5. Conserved semen could be used later if the dogs did not develop DCM, and more litters could be permitted for dogs in whose cases both parents or all grandparents had normal hearts at over 8 years of age. Heart testing results should be stored in a central database and made publicly available. Based on such data, simultaneous estimation of breeding values and genotype probabilities can be expected to be an effective tool in breeding against the disease (Vollmar, Fox et al. 2004).

The German Sighthound Club (DWZRV), which is responsible for Irish Wolfhound breeding in Germany, has introduced mandatory heart testing for dogs intended for breeding in 1999 and regularly publishes the results in its magazine (Anonymous 2005 a).

3.4 Osteogenic Sarcoma (OS)

3.4.1 Description

Osteogenic sarcoma is a highly aggressive primary tumour of the skeletal bones that occurs frequently in middle-aged large dogs, including Irish Wolfhounds. The metaphyses of the long limb bones are most frequently affected (Suter and Niemand 2001 b).

3.4.1.1 Pathophysiology

While the exact cause of OS is often unknown, it can occur where chronic irritation of the bone took place, e.g. osteomyelitis, unstable fractures, old fracture sites or around metallic implants. Genetically, several related tumour suppressor gene defects have been described in canine OS (van Leeuwen, Cornelisse et al. 1997; Johnson, Couto et al. 1998; Ferracini, Angelini et al. 2000; Levine, Forest et al. 2002). On the molecular level, the forming of cancer is a multi-step process involving DNA damage (either inherited or environmental), expression of growth promoters (pre-cancerous phase) and finally accumulation of further genetic changes, leading to increased malignancy (Ruttemann 2005).

OS cells are poorly differentiated, mesenchymal in nature and produce osteoid, bone substance and, occasionally, cartilaginous tissue. The tumour is characterised by an aggressive local osteolysis, periosteal reaction with the formation of new bone tissue and more or less pronounced soft tissue swelling. Micro-metastases occur early in the course of the disease; the most common sites being the lungs and other bones. Over 90% of affected individuals may have microscopic lung metastases at the time of diagnosis (Chun and Morrison 2004). Osteolysis can eventually lead to pathological fractures of the affected bone (Suter and Niemand 2001 b).

3.4.1.2 Symptoms

OS can remain without symptoms for some time and then gradually or suddenly cause various degrees of lameness, the development of which can be combined with an actual or perceived injury to the limb in question. Symptoms of manifest OS include lameness and strong pain upon palpation. A swelling is not obligatory and usually only easily discernable where the bone is not covered by muscle (Suter and

Niemand 2001 b). The most frequent locations are reported to be "far from the elbow, close to the knee" (Chun and Morrison 2004).

3.4.1.3 Diagnosis

Every metaphysical swelling in middle-aged large dogs should be considered potentially tumorous until this assumption is disproved (Suter and Niemand 2001 b). Radiographic signs include a combination of bone lysis and proliferation, which can lead to the characteristic "sunburst" pattern (Kramer, Latimer et al. 2003). As opposed to benign changes (osteomyelitis), there is no sclerotic demarcation line between the lesion and healthy bone tissue. Marked soft tissue swelling is also common (Suter and Niemand 2001 b; Chun and Morrison 2004).

Pulmonary metastases are often invisible at the time of diagnosis, but as stated above, it is very probable that micro-metastases are already present in dogs with manifest clinical signs of OS despite this. Nevertheless, thoracic radiographs (three views) should always been taken when OS is suspected (Chun and Morrison 2004).

It is also possible, although unusual to additionally do CT or scintigraphic bone scans to diagnose OS. CT is more sensitive at detecting early bone lysis, while scintigraphy may be useful for identifying metastatic disease at an earlier stage than X-rays. The latter procedure will not distinguish between sites of previous trauma or inflammation and metastases, however (Chun and Morrison 2004).

Laboratory findings are absent or non-specific, but it seems that an increased AP level is associated with a poorer prognosis (Chun and Morrison 2004).

The gold standard for diagnosis is a tumour biopsy. Given that different tumour types react differently to different therapy protocols and have varying prognoses, it should be considered if a specific therapy is planned. Multiple core biopsies using a Jamshidi needle may be necessary for a definite diagnosis though (Suter and Niemand 2001 b; Kramer, Latimer et al. 2003; Chun and Morrison 2004). Several personal communications from owners suggest that the procedure may not be well tolerated in Wolfhounds though.

3.4.1.4 Therapy

Standard therapy is amputation, which can be combined with an adjuvant platinum- (current standard of care) or platinum/doxorubicin-based chemotherapy protocol. As an alternative to amputation, limb-sparing surgical techniques may be attempted in case of distal radial lesions (Suter and Niemand 2001 b; Chun and Morrison 2004; Chun, Garrett et al. 2005). To assess how well a patient is going to tolerate amputation, it is advisable to bandage the affected leg against the body and observe the coping reaction for some time.

Palliative radiation protocols can be used to reduce pain and associated lameness and have been reported to be effective in over 70% of cases. They can also be combined with chemotherapy (Suter and Niemand 2001 b). It is also possible to limit palliative treatment to pain control with NSAIDs and/or fentanyl patches, although this should be limited to cases where no macroscopic metastases are evident (Suter and Niemand 2001 b).

Recently, the bisphosphonate drugs alendronate (Tomlin, Sturgeon et al. 2000; Farese, Ashton et al. 2004) and pamidronate (Ashton, Farese et al. 2005; Fan, de Lorimier et al. 2005) have shown some promising results in inhibiting the growth of canine osteosarcoma both in vitro and in vivo. Bisphosphonates are analogues of endogenous pyrophosphate, which is a naturally occurring inhibitor of bone metabolism. They have the potential to inhibit the osteolytic process and thus to reduce the pain associated with bone lesions through the inhibition of osteoclast activity.

Because of the small number of examined cases in the quoted publications, further research on this treatment option is necessary. The author is aware of one currently ongoing study on the subject (Dernell et al., in progress), in which Wolfhounds are treated with 40 mg of alendronate orally once per day or 70 mg every other day. No results have been released as of yet (August 2009).

3.4.1.5 Prognosis

OS has a generally poor prognosis and will usually result in the animal's death. In a population of 400'000 insured Swedish dogs (all breeds), median survival time of dogs with OS who survived the day of diagnosis was 56 days; in dogs who survived more than 30 days after diagnosis, median survival time was 274 days. (Egenvall, Nodtvedt et al. 2007). The authors conclude that this is due to the fact that a relatively high percentage of Swedish dogs diagnosed with OS receive no treatment other than palliative analgesics, and that the longer-surviving dogs likely received some form of additional treatment.

According to another source, the median survival time with palliative treatment alone (amputation without chemotherapy; pain control; palliative radiotherapy) is reported to be four months. The combination of surgery and chemotherapy increases median survival to around 10 months (Chun and Morrison 2004). There is only a small amount of published data on the life-prolonging properties of bisphosphonates, but survival was reported to be 10 and 12 months respectively in two cases treated with alendronate (Tomlin, Sturgeon et al. 2000).

3.4.2 Epizootology

In past studies of causes of death in Wolfhounds, OS was found to be responsible for between 21% (Bernardi 1986) and 24% (Prokopenko 1998) of deaths. In Bernardi's data, sex distribution of OS was almost equal, with 49.2% males and 50.8% females, while mean age at death was 6.6 years.

There are several numbers on odds ratios available: One study found Irish Wolfhounds to have an OR of 27.5 as compared to the overall dog population (Dorn 2002), whereas another found an OR of 20.7 as compared to German Shepherd dogs (Ru, Terracini et al. 1998). A study on insured Irish Wolfhounds from Sweden (Egenvall, Nodtvedt et al. 2007) found 23 cases in the study's 2'316 dog years at risk, which corresponds to a rate of 99 cases per 10'000 dog years at risk in a population of dogs aged 10 years and under. The average incidence in the population was 5.5 cases per 10'000 dog years at risk (OR = 18). Irish Wolfhounds had the highest risk of all breeds considered. Median age at diagnosis in the breed was 6.6 years.

However, the authors also remark that a comparably large percentage of OS in the overall dog population occur after 10 years of age, which, given the Irish Wolfhound's generally low life expectancy, may represent a bias when comparing OS incidence between breeds.

Castration has been described as a risk factor for developing OS (Priester and McKay 1980; Ru, Terracini et al. 1998; Cooley, Beranek et al. 2002). In this study, this could be reproduced in males only during re-evaluation of the Bernardi/Prokopenko data, in which information on castration status was available (see chapter 5.1.5.2). In the latter two quoted studies, it was hypothesised that the underlying mechanism may be associated with a longer bone growth period in castrated animals, whose growth plates close at a later age than those of intact animals.

Across all breeds, female dogs have been reported to be at a lower risk for osteosarcoma than males (Egenvall, Nodtvedt et al. 2007); however, this could not be reproduced in the study at hand, which found an increased risk in castrated males only as explained above.

3.4.3 Heredity and Control Measures

Despite the fact that the incidence of OS varies strongly between different dog breeds, and although familial predispositions have been reported in the species (Bech-Nielsen, Haskins et al. 1978), relatively little is known about its underlying hereditary mechanisms. Involvement of mutations of the p53 tumour suppressor gene has been described, as have changes in several proto-oncogenes (van Leeuwen, Cornelisse et al. 1997; Johnson, Couto et al. 1998; Mendoza, Konishi et al. 1998; Ferracini, Angelini et al. 2000; Meyer, Murua Escobar et al. 2004). Furthermore, a strong familial OS predisposition has recently been discovered in the Scottish Deerhound (Hauck, personal communication).

Hereditary cancers are unlikely to be mediated by defective proto-oncogenes, since their expression would interfere with the development of the embryo. On the other hand, a hereditary cancer caused by a germ line mutation of a tumour suppressor gene can be expected to follow a dominant pattern of inheritance, combined with incomplete penetrance (environmental interaction and other modulating factors) and embryonic death (lethal factor) in homozygous individuals. However, there are other possible mechanisms of hereditary cancer transmission as well, which can be transmitted through mutations in different modulator genes (Ruttemann 2005).

Initial research on Osteosarcoma in Scottish Deerhounds (a breed closely related to the Irish Wolfhound) at the Universities of North Carolina and Tennessee indicated a simple autosomal recessive mode of inheritance, but this has been shown to be too simple an approach in the meantime (Hauck, personal communication).

Given the currently available literature, it is realistic to assume a hereditary component of the disease, the exact nature of which remains unknown for the time being. It therefore seems reasonable not to breed individuals diagnosed with the disease. Further research concerning the mode of inheritance is needed to determine more precise breeding recommendations for relatives of affected animals. In the meantime, estimated breeding values could be a useful tool for selection.

Additionally, given the risk association with male castration, it is recommended not to routinely castrate male Irish Wolfhounds. If the owner insists to have the procedure performed, it should at least be postponed until after the end of the growth period. The owner should be informed that the correlation with the longer growth period in castrated males is hypothetical, and that there may still be an increase in OS risk even if the procedure is performed after the completion of growth.

3.5 Gastric Dilation and Volvulus (GDV)

3.5.1 Description

Gastric Dilation and Volvulus is the dilation and torsion of the stomach and spleen, leading to blood sequestration, necrosis, distributive shock and often death. Large, deep-chested dog breeds from age 2 to 3 upwards are at an increased risk (Glickman, Glickman et al. 2000 b; Suter and Niemand 2001 c; Waschak and Jergens 2004).

3.5.1.1 Pathophysiology

Acute gastric dilation occurs following copious feeding and/or stress. It can be due to both excessive filling of the stomach and decreased motility, which compromises the natural stomach emptying mechanism. The dilation can be aggravated through aerophagy, the release of CO_2 due to the reaction of HCl with bicarbonate (saliva/duodenal reflux) and the release of gases due to fermentation. Subsequently, the greater curvature over-expands and thus dislocates the pylorus, leading to the actual torsion (usually clockwise when watched from behind), which blocks both the entry and the exit of the stomach. Due to its close anatomical association with the stomach, the spleen is also included in the torsion.

As more and more gas is produced, the stomach continues to expand, compressing both the V. cava caudalis and the V. Porta, thereby leading to blood sequestration in the caudal body. The splenic veins are also blocked, which leads to concurrent blood sequestration into the spleen, all of which contributes to distributive shock. Furthermore, the expanding stomach interferes with diaphragm movement, decreasing respiratory volume. The spleen and stomach walls can become necrotic, allowing toxins to pass into the blood and causing reperfusion injury if the condition is treated.

Decreased cardiac output is accentuated by insufficient lung function due to lung compression by the dilated stomach, leading to progressive systemic hypoxia, distributive shock and subsequent death (Suter and Niemand 2001 c; Waschak and Jergens 2004).

3.5.1.2 Symptoms

GDV is most frequently observed in the evening or during the night, usually following copious feeding. Symptoms include restlessness, unsuccessful attempts to vomit and characteristic abdominal swelling in combination with a tympanic percussion sound.

Symptoms of shock rapidly develop and lead to collapse and death if left untreated (Suter and Niemand 2001 c; Waschak and Jergens 2004).

3.5.1.3 Diagnosis

The history and clinical presentation of GDV cases is usually fairly characteristic of the disease. If the state of the patient allows for an X-ray to be taken (right lateral recumbency), torsion can be differentiated from simple dilation using this method. The dilated and torsed stomach usually exhibits the classical "double bubble" pattern (Waschak and Jergens 2004).

3.5.1.4 Therapy

Treatment only has a chance if action is taken promptly and purposefully. If the first response practice is not equipped to perform an emergency operation, it is crucial to make a rapid diagnosis and initiate emergency patient stabilisation before referring the patient to an appropriately equipped clinic.

Emergency stabilisation consists of decompression and shock treatment. At first, initial decompression is achieved through percutaneous punction with a 1.2 mm (18 Gauge) needle through the left flank. The needle is then attached to a suction pump, and suction is continued until operation in order to relieve the pressure on the main veins and diaphragm.

Alternatively, it is possible to try to achieve decompression through a thick oesophageal probe in the standing, non-sedated or mildly sedated dog (Suter and Niemand 2001 c; Waschak and Jergens 2004). This is reported to be rarely successful due to the blocked antrum, although failure to reach the stomach can be considered diagnostic for complete torsion.

Second, shock treatment should be initiated by putting an i.v. catheter into the cephalic vein (alternatively, catheters can be put into both cephalic veins to achieve faster fluid administration) and applying 7 ml/kg of a plasma expander, mixed with 20 ml/kg of Ringer lactate. 4 mg/kg each of gentamycin and dexamethasone can also be added. Using a caudal vein (e.g. the V. saphena) for the infusion is contraindicated, given that the caudal caval vein is compressed by the dilated stomach (Suter and Niemand 2001 c).

It should be noted that there is some controversy regarding the order in which decompression and fluid therapy should be initiated. For example, (Waschak and Jergens 2004) find it preferable to attempt decompression only after the initiation of fluid therapy.

After stabilisation of the patient is achieved, surgical decompression, reposition and gastropexy should be undertaken in an adequately equipped clinic. If the patient fails to respond to stabilisation measures, surgery should be initiated as quickly as possible (Waschak and Jergens 2004). Several surgical techniques have been described in the literature. The following technique is taken from (Suter and Niemand 2001 c):

Standard surgical preparation (shaving, washing, initial disinfection etc.) is performed on the standing animal under continuous infusion and decompression. Inhalation anaesthesia (pure O_2) is combined with neuroleptanalgesia (cave: drugs that may exacerbate hypovolaemia are counterindicated, e.g. acepromazine). The dog is placed in dorsal recumbency, and the peritoneum opened in the linea alba from the xiphoid to a point caudal of the umbilicus. The stomach is exposed and advanced using two supramide filaments. Wet swabs are placed around the wound to seal off the peritoneum, and a 7 cm incision is made into the larger curvature. The contents of the stomach are removed using a suction pump. The tube should have an internal diameter between 2.5 and 4 cm, depending on the consistence of the ingesta. 30 to 50 (!) active coal tablets are placed into the stomach, and the wound is then closed using a double stomach suture technique. The supramide filaments are removed, and the operation field is cleaned thoroughly and then closed.

To achieve retrotorsion, the duodenum descendens is identified (associated pancreatic lobe) and followed until the pylorus is reached. The stomach is then put back into its normal position through manipulation of the pylorus and antrum. The retrotorsed stomach is thoroughly examined for injured vessels and necrotic parts. Occasionally, it is necessary to invaginate necrotic parts through an invaginating suture. Partial gastrectomy at the larger curvature is rarely required.

The spleen is also thoroughly examined for injured vessels and thromboses and removed if necessary. Suter and Niemand (2001 c) additionally recommend performing a pyloric myotomy to facilitate stomach emptying.

Finally, a gastropexy is performed at the antrum and the peritoneum closed. It is considered malpractice not to include gastropexy in GDV surgery.

Postoperatively, Ringer lactate infusion should be continued for 24 h. 4 mg/kg of gentamycin and an antibiotic of the cephalosporin family should be added to prevent infection. Gastric acid should be reduced through the addition of cimetidine or ranitidine in order to prevent gastric ulceration. The heart should be monitored closely for 48 hours, and an ECG taken thrice a day. Occasional extrasystoles (due to toxaemia) are normal, but must be treated if they become frequent. For this purpose, flecainide acetate 2 mg/kg is given intravenously over 30 minutes, and 8 mg/kg/d are added to the infusion (Suter and Niemand 2001 c). Electrolyte supplementation is also often indicated (Waschak and Jergens 2004).

After 48 hours of fasting, feeding is started with small, multiple feedings of an easily digestible diet. Suter and Niemand (2001 c) recommend continuing feeding twice daily after an episode of GDV.

3.5.1.5 Prognosis

Fatality rates have been described to range from 15 to 24% (Glickman, Glickman et al. 2000 a). Possible complications include severe arrhythmias due to toxaemia, reperfusion injury, and ulceration and perforation of the stomach and ensuing peritonitis. Prognosis depends on the time passed between the occurrence of the first symptoms and the initiation of decompression and shock management. Without gastropexy, relapse rates have been described to be around 80%, while they decrease to 3-5% if gastropexy is used. Prognosis is good in dogs that survive the first three to four days post-operatively (Suter and Niemand 2001 c).

3.5.2 Epizootology

A prospective study of 177 Irish Wolfhounds, of which 10 developed GDV during the study period, found that the breed has a GDV incidence of 2.6% per year, 3.6% in males and 1.8% in females. The risk of GDV increased by approximately 20% per additional year of age (Glickman, Glickman et al. 2000 a). On a more general note, older, large and giant purebred dogs with a deep and narrow thorax were found to be at an increased risk (Burrows and Ignaszweski 1990).

Gastric Dilation Volvulus (GDV) accounted for 11.7% of reported deaths in Irish Wolfhounds (Bernardi 1986). The Hoflin survey found a similar number of 11.5% (Prokopenko 1998). As opposed to other breed-specific diseases, the comparatively low lethality of GDV makes it difficult to assess its incidence from death data as used in these studies as well as the study at hand.

The author hypothesises that to a certain extent, the basic laws of mechanics and inertia could also be contributing to the higher GDV incidence in large breed dogs: While the mass of the stomach increases cubically (proportional to its volume) as the dog's size increases, the strength of its gastric ligaments only increases quadratically (proportional to their cross-sectional area). Hence, the larger the dog grows, the less favourable the relation between stomach mass and ligament strength becomes.

3.5.3 Heredity and Control Measures

Having a first-degree relative (parent/sibling/offspring) affected with GDV has been associated with an increased GDV risk for a long time. In a recent prospective study, dogs that had at least one first-degree relative affected with GDV had an adjusted risk increase of 63%, indicating a hereditary component. This hereditary component may be partly mediated through the inheritance of a particular body shape or temperament (Glickman, Glickman et al. 2000 b).

The same study concludes that dogs with a first-degree relative with GDV should not be used for breeding, and that the incidence of the disease could be reduced by 60% using this approach. Using a proportional hazard risk model, the data also showed that a 14% overall decrease of GDV cases in the population could be reached by this selection approach (Glickman, Glickman et al. 2000 b).

3.6 Rhinitis/Bronchopneumonia Syndrome – PCD

3.6.1 Description

Rhinitis/Bronchopneumonia syndrome is a disease of the respiratory tract that usually affects Irish Wolfhound puppies from the time of birth. Other organs such as the cerebral ventricles, middle ear and male reproductive tract can also be affected. The syndrome was one of the earliest diseases described in the breed, at the time as probably viral in origin (Wilkinson 1969). Only recently has the link been made to the possible mechanisms of a hereditary immunodeficiency (Leisewitz, Spencer et al. 1997) and/or of hereditary Primary Ciliary Dyskinesia (Clercx, Reichler et al. 2003; Casal 2004).

3.6.1.1 Possible Pathophysiologies

Primary Ciliary Dyskinesia (PCD) is a disorder of the cilia found in the epithelium of the respiratory and reproductive tract (internal wall of the vasa deferentia and sperm flagella), as well as the auditory tubes, the cerebral ventricles and the oviducts. These cilia play an important role in mucociliary clearance and in the transport of germ cells through the reproductive tract. If their normal motility is impaired, this can lead to chronic infectious bronchopneumonia, secretory otitis media, hydrocephalus, and infertility (Edwards and Johnson 2004).

An alternative explanation would be that the syndrome is caused by a defect in the immune system, the nature of which is yet to be determined. This would lead to increased susceptibility to infection, resulting in the clinical signs seen in affected Irish Wolfhounds. In one study, a decreased lymphocyte response to blastogenic factors was reported in three affected Irish Wolfhounds (Leisewitz, Spencer et al. 1997). The validity of these findings has recently been questioned by arguing that very sick or dying dogs usually have a certain degree of abnormal immune responses as compared to healthy dogs (Casal 2004).

Given the available evidence for a hereditary base, the hypothesis of a viral infection (Wilkinson 1969) should be considered obsolete nowadays.

3.6.1.2 Symptoms

The condition occurs in young Irish Wolfhound puppies and is often apparent at birth. A watery nasal discharge is present, which turns purulent as secondary infection develops. As the infection progresses, bronchopneumonia develops, which, although responsive to antibiotics, is often recurrent and a common cause of death. Turbinate atrophy can also occur (Clercx, Reichler et al. 2003), and a persistent catarrhal vaginal or praeputial discharge has been recorded as a symptom in one study (Wilkinson 1969).

In some cases, hydrocephalus (Clercx, Reichler et al. 2003; Casal 2004) and otitis media (Clercx, Reichler et al. 2003) have also been reported, which would fit the expected picture of PCD. While no significant number of electron microscopic ciliary abnormalities were found by (Clercx, Reichler et al. 2003), unpublished data seem to suggest that there are abnormal ciliary beating patterns and electron microscopic ciliary abnormities in affected Wolfhounds (Casal 2004).

3.6.1.3 Diagnosis

The typical clinical history of recurrent non-contagious mucopurulent nasal discharge and bronchopneumonia that have been present since birth or shortly afterwards is fairly indicative of the syndrome. Thoracic radiography usually reveals features of chronic bronchopneumonia and sometimes bronchiectasis. Thickened, sclerotic tympanic bullæ (otitis media) and rhinoliths can also be present. Trans-tracheal lavage typically yields mucous to mucopurulent material that can be cytologically identified as a purulent exsudate. As a diagnostic test for PCD, tracheal mucous clearance can be measured using ^{99}Tc scintigraphy.

Differential diagnoses include recurrent aspiration pneumonia (e.g. caused by megaoesophagus or broncho-oesophagal fistula), chronic bronchopneumonia caused by resistant bacteria, chronic distemper, ehrlichiosis, fungal rhinitis, and nasal or tracheobronchial foreign bodies (Edwards and Johnson 2004).

3.6.1.4 Therapy

The therapeutic approach is symptomatic and consists of aggressive antibiotic treatment for bronchopneumonia, which should be based on bacterial culture and resistance analysis. The duration should vary depending on the severity of infection and the reaction of the individual dog, but it must be noted that continuous antibiotic therapy can often lead to colonisation with resistant bacteria. Acute episodes of bronchopneumonia may require oxygen therapy.

To improve mucociliary clearance, routine exercise is recommended, which can be combined with steam inhalation therapy. Daily positioning of the patient in dorsal recumbency has been recommended to promote drainage of mucus from the airways and thus expectoration (Edwards and Johnson 2004).

3.6.1.5 Prognosis

The disease is incurable, but survival times are highly variable. The longest recorded survival time was found in an Irish Wolfhound male who reached 8 years of age and died of unrelated causes (Clercx, Reichler et al. 2003). Prognosis is considerably worse in patients showing signs at less than one year of age, where chronic bronchopneumonia can have life-threatening periodical exacerbations (Edwards and Johnson 2004).

Appropriate antibiotic treatment and pulmonary physical therapy may prolong survival, but complications of chronic airway infection such as reactive systemic amyloidosis or cor pulmonale are possible. Nevertheless, some patients can still reach a normal lifespan if treated appropriately (Edwards and Johnson 2004).

3.6.2 Epizootology

No numbers on the incidence and prevalence of the syndrome in Irish Wolfhounds have been published in the veterinary literature. However, in one study, all examined disease cases belong to six bloodlines, and all of these dogs share common ancestors (Clercx, Reichler et al. 2003). It is thus probable that the syndrome is still limited to certain families within the Wolfhound population, although the increasing degree of outcrossing could change this in the future.

3.6.3 Heredity and Control Measures

While Wilkison (1969) favoured a viral aetiology over a hereditary base for the disease, both Leisewitz, Spencer et al. (1997) and Clercx, Reichler et al. (2003) offer evidence for a hereditary disease. As of today, the mode of inheritance is thought to follow a simple autosomal recessive pattern. No DNA markers are available as of yet, but there is an ongoing international research project to identify one at the universities of Zurich and Pennsylvania (Casal 2004; Casal and Henthorn 2008).

No concrete breeding recommendations are given in the literature, although in such cases, it is generally recommended not to breed the carriers identified through their production of affected offspring, and not to breed the probable carriers, i.e. full siblings of affected individuals. Breeding affected males is impossible due to their infertility in the case of PCD, and breeding affected females is, of course, strongly discouraged.

3.7 Juvenile Fibrocartilaginous Embolism (FCE)

3.7.1 Description

Fibrocartilaginous embolism is an infarction of the spinal marrow that occurs in juvenile Irish Wolfhounds. This age group is atypical, since the disease is usually reported to be a problem of dogs aged 3-5 years (Junker, van den Ingh et al. 2000; Sisson and Parent 2004). The occurrence of FCE in juvenile Wolfhounds (two individuals aged 16 and 19 weeks) was first reported in the literature in 1993 (Dyce and Houlton 1993).

3.7.1.1 Pathophysiology

The embolism is caused by cartilaginous material from the nucleus pulposus of the intervertebral discs that becomes entrapped in the blood vessels leading to the spinal marrow. This leads to spinal infarction, neuromalacia and, consequently, to both sensory and motoric neurological deficits.

The exact mechanism through which the cartilaginous material can enter the bloodstream is unknown. It is hypothesised that chronic stress injury to the intervertebral discs can lead to Hansen type II disc degeneration, leading to inflammatory angiogenesis in the annulus fibrosus. Trauma and/or exercise may then increase intradiscal pressure, leading to insudation of the nucleus pulposus into the inflamed annulus and thus into the newly formed blood vessels (Sisson and Parent 2004).

However, this mechanism cannot explain FCE in juvenile animals, since Hansen type II degeneration has only been found in adult dogs. It is thus hypothesised that the discrepancy between the rapid increase in weight and slow skeletal ossification in Wolfhounds may lead to increased pressure on the intervertebral discs. This could press nucleus pulposus material into the annulus fibrosus, which is still well-vascularised in juvenile animals (Junker, van den Ingh et al. 2000).

3.7.1.2 Symptoms

The main clinical manifestation of FCE is abnormal locomotion, which can range from discrete ataxia to complete tetraplegia. The onset of symptoms is acute, ranging from seconds to hours, but the condition should be stable within 12 to 24 hours. There is often an associated history of trauma and/or exercise, which can be as discrete as playing or a short walk. Affected puppies usually cry in pain at the time of onset, but this pain subsides within minutes to (at most) a few hours (Sisson and Parent 2004).

3.7.1.3 Diagnosis

The definite diagnosis of FCE can only be made post mortem through histopathological examination of the spinal chord, combined with special staining techniques to demonstrate the presence of cartilaginous material inside the medullary blood vessels (Junker, van den Ingh et al. 2000). Nevertheless, FCE can be strongly suspected in vivo if the following diagnostic criteria are met:

Neurological examination reveals spinal injury of widely varying location and severity. Diagnostic criteria include acute onset, absence of pain, usually (though not always) asymmetrical neurological signs, a history of trauma and/or exercise shortly before the onset, and non-progressive symptoms after 12-24 hours at most. If the symptoms continue to progress after this period, other causes of neuromalacia should be considered.

Spinal radiographs are usually normal. Myelography often shows focal intramedullary swelling in the acute stage. Later on, it can be normal or indicate focal medullary atrophy. MRI is currently the best available diagnostic technique, with the responsible disc showing decreased and the infarcted medullary area showing increased signal intensity on T2 images. However, its limited availability and the need for fast action in acute cases can limit its practical use.

Furthermore, a cerebrospinal fluid analysis can be performed. In the acute stage, it may show a high RBC and a mildly increased neutrophile count; later on, only mildly elevated protein levels may be observed. Normal results are also possible at all stages, however.

Differential diagnoses include other forms of spinal injury such as fractures and luxations, which are usually associated with pain and visible on a spinal radiography; or spinal tumours (Vaughan-Scott, Goldin et al. 1999), where signs can be expected to be slowly progressive rather than acute (also see chapter 3.12.8). Furthermore, medullary haemorrhage due to ingestion of rodenticides, thrombocytopenia or DIC should be considered and excluded through a haematological exam. Last, focal myelitis is also a possibility, but can be differentiated by its progressive symptoms and characteristic changes in the cerebrospinal fluid (Sisson and Parent 2004).

Sex	Age (wks)	Trauma?	Clinical Diagnosis	Pathology
m	9	yes (play)	Tetraparesis/-plegia; problem C1-C6	FCE C5-C7
m	12.5	yes (slid)	Monoparesis; left hind limb	FCE T1-T7
m	8	unknown	Hemiparesis/-plegia	FCE C6-C7
m	10	unknown	Hemiparesis	FCE C5-T3
f	8	no	Paresis posterior	FCE
m	11	no	Monoparesis/-plegia; left hind limb	recovered
m	10	yes (walk)	Monoparesis; left hind limb	recovered
m	11	no	Paresis posterior; problem T2-L3	recovered

Table 3.6: Summary of clinical presentation data from 8 Irish Wolfhound pups diagnosed with or suspected of FCE over a 16 month period between 1996 and 1997 at Utrecht university; taken from (Junker, van den Ingh et al. 2000). Note that the definition of "trauma" is to be interpreted generously, which could interfere with the cases where no trauma was reported.

3.7.1.4 Therapy

Methylprednisolone sodium succinate has been reported to be beneficial if treatment is initiated within the first 8 hours after the onset of symptoms. 30 mg/kg are given i.v. as an initial dose, followed by 15 mg/kg after 2 and 6 hours and then every 6 hours over a total period of 24-48 hours. Each injection should be given slowly, over 10 to 15 minutes in order to prevent vomiting. Treatment should not be continued for more than 48 hours, since no additional benefits have been shown and the risk of gastrointestinal ulceration is greatly increased with more prolonged use. NSAIDs are counterindicated, since their combination with methylprednisolone succinate also increases adverse effects. A high-fibre diet can be given in order to reduce the risk of gastrointestinal ulceration.

Recumbent patients should be kept on a soft surface and turned frequently in order to prevent the formation of decubitus ulcers. All patients should be assisted and encouraged to walk as soon as possible (hydrotherapy being a very valuable option in these cases). Neurological examination should be repeated frequently during the first 12 to 24 hours in order to detect a possible progression of symptoms. It should then be repeated after 2, 3 and 4 weeks in order to document the further clinical course, which is relevant for the prognosis (see below).

In case of urinary incontinence, urinalysis and bacterial culture should be performed to identify a possible infection (Sisson and Parent 2004).

3.7.1.5 Prognosis

Intact pain perception and upper motor neuron signs usually indicate a good prognosis for marked improvement, whereas the complete loss of pain perception is indicative of a poor prognosis. Areflexia of limbs or sphincters gives the dog almost no chance of recovery, while functional recovery is common if purposeful movements and reflexes are merely reduced – although some degree of permanent deficit is likely in these cases.

A progression of the clinical signs from upper to lower motor neuron and an enlarging area of sensory loss suggest the presence of progressive neuromalacia and indicate a hopeless prognosis. Euthanasia should be considered in these cases.

Marked changes in neurological status are unlikely to occur during the first 14 days after the onset of symptoms. Most improvement can be expected to occur between days 21 and 42. If no improvement is seen after 21 to 30 days, recovery becomes highly unlikely (Sisson and Parent 2004).

3.7.2 Epizootology

There are no published numbers concerning incidence and prevalence of juvenile FCE in Irish Wolfhounds in the veterinary literature. The high number of FCE puppies (8 during a period of 16 months) treated at Utrecht University could be coincidental, but the authors state that anecdotal evidence from dog breeder journals suggests that FCE is a common occurrence in juvenile Irish Wolfhounds. The author of the study at hand is also aware of several probable FCE cases from the UK and the US.

Furthermore, the Utrecht cases also show an overrepresentation of males, but again, the number of cases is too low to draw a definite conclusion (Junker, van den Ingh et al. 2000). However, with a H_0 of equal gender distribution, a binomial test of table 3.6 results in a $P=0.034$ (two-tailed $z=-2.12$)

3.7.3 Heredity and Control Measures

In the Utrecht cases presented in table 3.6, two dogs (numbers 2 and 6) came from the same litter, and their mother was reported to have had transient neurological problems at the same age as her pups. The breeder of case 5 reported that he had had four similar cases in the same line. While such anecdotal evidence is insufficient as exact proof, it is an indication that there may well be a hereditary component in the development of FCE in Irish Wolfhounds, the nature of which remains yet to be determined (Junker, van den Ingh et al. 2000). On this base, it is probably indicated not to use affected individuals for breeding, but further research is necessary to make more specific recommendations.

3.8 Epilepsy

3.8.1 Description

Epilepsy is a brain disorder that is characterised by recurrent seizures in the absence of a concurrent brain lesion. While the brain appears to be structurally normal, there are functional abnormalities that periodically result in disorganized neuronal discharge patterns (Parent 2004). The disease has been shown to be hereditary in Wolfhounds (Casal, Munuve et al. 2006).

3.8.1.1 Pathophysiology

The exact pathophysiological mechanisms of epilepsy are unknown. It has been hypothesised that there may be chemical imbalances in the brain (e.g. a genetic defect in the neuronal membranes or in neurotransmitter function) or that an animal may have an intrinsic propensity to have seizures. The existence of different disease mechanisms in different breeds is very likely (Thomas 1994; Parent 2004).

3.8.1.2 Symptoms

Since epileptic dogs do not usually show clinical abnormalities at the time of presentation, an extensive and detailed history must be taken from the owner (Thomas 1994). Irish Wolfhounds affected with epilepsy usually exhibit grand mal seizures (Casal, Munuve et al. 2006), which can include stiffness, chomping or clenching of the jaw, vocalisation, defaecation and urination, profuse salivation, and paddling with all four limbs. Post-seizure behaviour can be characterised by periods of confusion and disorientation, neurological deficits, aimless and compulsive blind pacing, and frequently polyuria and polydipsia. Recovery time after the end of a seizure varies – it may be instant, but may also take up to 24 hours (Parent 2004).

3.8.1.3 Diagnosis

The diagnosis of epilepsy is essentially reached through the exclusion of any other underlying disease. The owner should be asked about illnesses or trauma, possibilities for poisoning, and vaccination history. A full neurological exam should also be performed, but should be repeated at a later time if generalised abnormalities are detected soon after a seizure. Dogs with idiopathic epilepsy do not have inter-ictal neurological deficits (Thomas 1994).

Differential diagnoses include seizures secondary to Portosystemic shunt (see chapter 3.2), especially in younger animals; toxicity; structural brain disease including tumours or scarring; and seizures secondary to other systemic disease processes. A full laboratory workup is indicated to detect such possible changes. Further possibilities include radiography, CT or MRI, and cerebrospinal fluid analysis, depending on what other causes are suspected (Parent 2004).

3.8.1.4 Therapy

Treatment should be initiated after the second generalised seizure, if there are acute cluster seizures or status epilepticus. The latter two states should be addressed early and aggressively.

Phenobarbital is the drug of first choice in the treatment of canine epilepsy. The goal is to reach a serum level of 100-120 µg/ml in the steady state, which takes between 12 and 15 days to reach.

In dogs with hepatic insufficiency or insufficient reaction to phenobarbital alone, potassium bromide (KBr) can also be used. Serum levels in the steady state should be between 1.2 and 1.6 mg/ml

3.8.1.5 Prognosis

The life expectancy of Irish Wolfhounds affected with epilepsy is reduced by about two years (Casal, Munuve et al. 2006). This finding should be interpreted with caution, however, since in the quoted study, the presented survival data of epileptic Wolfhounds are likely tainted with right censored data (see 3.1.1.3) and then compared to the Bernardi data (see 3.1.3.1), which has been shown to also be subject to this bias in the present study (Urfer and Steiger 2006).

In a population of n=126 epileptic Irish Wolfhounds, 76 (60.3%) died as a direct result of the disease. These seizure-related deaths were classified as death during seizure (16.1%), euthanasia due to uncontrolled seizures (65.8%), phenobarbital hepatotoxicity (6.6%), aspiration during seizure and subsequent fatal pneumonia (6.6%), and euthanasia due to non-recovery after a seizure (3.9%). The other 50 dogs (39.7%) died from unrelated causes. Median survival time after the first seizure did not vary significantly between different ages at onset (Casal, Munuve et al. 2006) as reproduced in figure 3.2 below. Again, these survival data are right censored and thus likely too low.

The lack of a significant difference in survival time after the first seizure is somewhat surprising when considering the considerable number of dogs who had their first seizure at a relatively advanced age (also see figure 3.3 below). Given the results for life expectancy in the study at hand, as well as in other studies, one would have presumed that the survival in dogs diagnosed at a more advanced age would have a shorter survival time due to unrelated causes of death.

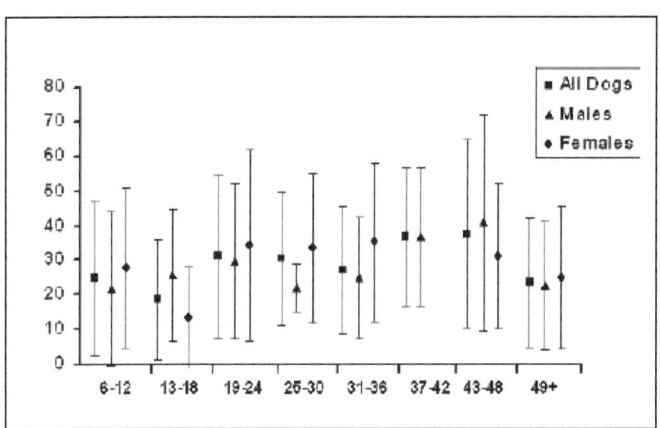

Figure 3.2: Survival times after first seizure by age at onset, reproduced from Casal, Munuve et al. (2006). X: Age at first seizure; Y: Survival time after first seizure. All times are in months. There are no significant (P>0.05) differences between groups.

3.8.2 Epizootology

An epilepsy incidence of 18.7% was described in a group of n=796 related Irish Wolfhounds from 120 litters (Casal, Munuve et al. 2006). This figure is unlikely to be representative of the whole population, however, since only 23 of these dogs came from litters (n=5) that were free of epilepsy, even though they were born to parents who had both produced affected offspring in other matings.

Mean ± SD age at onset was 27.6 ± 16.8 months in females and 33.9 ± 18.5 months in males. The overall age ranges for seizure onset were 6 to 84 months in females and 6 to 107 months in males. Significantly more dogs had their first seizure before 3 years of age than after 3 years of age (P<0.05), with 87% of females, but only 67% of males having their first seizure before this age. Overall, a male-to-female ratio of 1:0.6 was found, which differed significantly from the overall population (P=0.01). However, there were no significant gender differences at 30 months and even 3 years of age. A summary of age distributions at the time of first seizure is reproduced in figure 3.3

Additionally, Casal, Munuve et al. (2006) also reported that in 23 litters with multiple affected individuals, the onset of seizures in littermates occurred within 12 months of each other, apart from 7 litters in which 1 dog each had its first seizure later in life. There also was one case of a repeat litter, where the age of onset of the four affected individuals (two per litter) covered a range of 3 years.

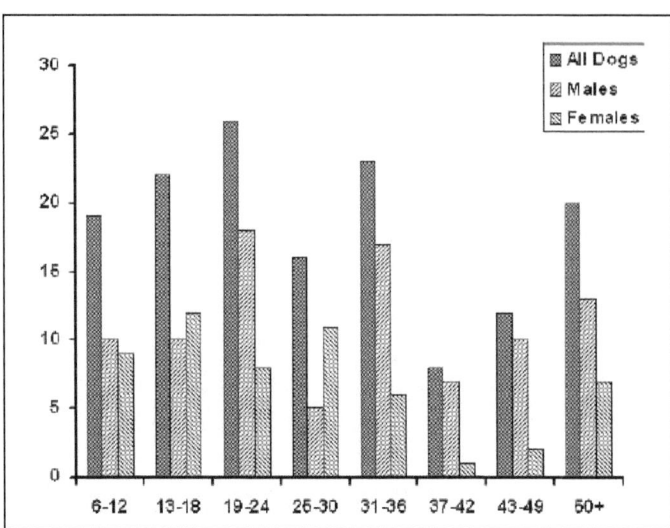

Fig. 3.3: Numbers of dogs of different ages at first seizure, reproduced from Casal, Munuve et al. (2006). X: age in months; Y: number of dogs. Significant differences (P<0.05) were found between females of the 37-49 months groups and the rest of the population, as well as between males and females for both the 37-42 and the 43-49 months group.

3.8.3 Heredity and Control Measures

In the previously mentioned related population with an epilepsy incidence of 18.7%, it was found that most affected individuals (143 dogs from 112 litters) were the offspring of clinically healthy parents. Only 3 affected dogs had an affected parent. Segregation ratio and heritability (h^2) were then calculated based on litters with healthy parents where medical records were available for all littermates. This resulted in a h^2 value of 0.87 and an estimated segregation ratio of 0.083 ± 0.0001. In contrast to all but two other studies on canine epilepsy, male Wolfhounds were found to be at an increased risk. However, if only seizure cases of dogs under 3 years were taken into account, there was no sex predilection present. No correlation between inbreeding and age at first seizure was found.

The fact that most affected Wolfhounds had healthy parents indicates a recessive mode of inheritance, and the h^2 >0.5 suggests the presence of a major gene. However, a segregation ratio <0.25 indicates that at the same time, a fully penetrant autosomal recessive inheritance is unlikely. The increased risk in older males could either indicate a sex-modifier gene, the presence of misdiagnosed primary conditions in the older animals, or that the seizures first appearing in dogs over 3 years of age have an independent mode of inheritance. Given that 55 out of 56 affected females were born to normal sires, an X-linked recessive inheritance is not likely, although the increased risk for males would still suggest such a model.

It was concluded that epilepsy in Irish Wolfhounds is highly heritable, but genetically complex. The suggested inheritance model for all affected dogs was an incompletely penetrant recessive trait with a sex predilection for older males (Casal, Munuve et al. 2006).

The authors of the quoted study chose not to provide practical breeding suggestions to control epilepsy in Irish Wolfhounds, but stress the need for the development of a genetic test. More recently, they have released preliminary results stating that several promising SNPs on chromosome 22 are under investigation (Casal, Werner et al. 2009). Other studies on diseases with complex modes of inheritance suggest that such diseases can be successfully addressed through estimated breeding values as long as no DNA-based testing is available (van Hagen, Janss et al. 2004).

3.9 Osteochondrosis (OC)

Osteochondrosis is an orthopaedic problem that is commonly encountered in growing dogs. While there are no studies dealing with the condition in Irish Wolfhounds specifically, the breed is fast-growing and thus at a higher risk to develop the disease than the average dog population (Dorn 2002; Schwarz and Shires 2004 a).

3.9.1 Description

OC can manifest itself in several forms, which can generally be divided into joint and growth plate problems. It is characterised by problems in the enchondral ossification process, leading to an excessive retention of cartilage that can lead to further complications (Schwarz and Shires 2004 a).

3.9.1.1 Pathophysiology

Chondrocytes of the immature joint and/or growth plate cartilage fail to differentiate normally, which interferes with the normal process of enchondral ossification during skeletal growing. Since the cartilage continues to grow without being replaced by bone, this leads to regions with excessively thick cartilage, which is less resistant to mechanical stress than bone.

Since joint cartilage nutrition is maintained through synovial diffusion, a thickening of joint cartilage results in an impaired metabolism which itself leads to degeneration and necrosis of the poorly supplied cells. This causes further weakening of the cartilage and may progress to the formation of a free cartilage flap inside the joint (Osteochondritis dissecans – OCD).

Retention of cartilage in growth plates does not usually cause necrosis, but may result in asymmetric growth (Schwarz and Shires 2004 a). Some authors hypothesise that this process is also involved in the development of certain variants of elbow dysplasia (ED), which are summarised under "short radius" or "short ulna" syndrome and subsequent fracture of the anconeal or coronoid processes (Schawalder 1997).

3.9.1.2 Symptoms

Symptoms depend on the affected joint(s) and/or growth plate(s), as well as on the presence of concurrent degenerative joint disease (DJD). A history of lameness of varying degrees that becomes worse after exercise is usually present; the patient may put little weight on the affected limb (Schwarz and Shires 2004 a).

3.9.1.3 Diagnosis

During orthopaedic examination, pain can usually be provoked by flexion, extension or rotation of the affected joint. Joint effusion and capsular distension may also be present. Muscle atrophy can develop in certain cases.

Radiography is the main means of diagnosis and usually shows sclerosis of the underlying bone (may be discrete), exostostoses and incongruencies depending on the affected joint. Comparison with the contralateral joint can also be useful for diagnosis.

Synovial fluid analysis shows decreased viscosity and >10'000 nucleated cells per µl, of which >90% should be mononuclear. OCD lesions can also be identified and removed during arthroscopy.

Differential diagnoses include trauma and/or intra-articular fractures, septic arthritis, panosteitis, hypertrophic osteodystrophy, avulsion or calcification of flexor muscles in elbow dysplasia, and synovial cell tumours. These can usually be differentiated through radiography and synovial fluid analysis (Schwarz and Shires 2004 a).

3.9.1.4 Therapy

Uncomplicated articular OC is not directly treatable. Affected dogs should receive exercise restriction and reduced caloric intake to promote slower growth. Furthermore, NSAIDs can be given for pain control (may interfere with exercise restriction), and chondroprotective drugs such as glycosaminoglycanes, glucosamine, or chondroitin sulphate may be given to prevent further damage and degeneration of cartilage (Schwarz and Shires 2004 a).

OCD should be addressed surgically by removal of the lose cartilage flap through arthrotomy or arthroscopy. Abrasion of the underlying bone to promote repair through fibrous cartilage formation is discussed controversially (Brunnberg, Burger et al. 2005).

Elbow dysplasia due to short radius/short ulna syndrome can be addressed through dynamic osteotomy in order to re-establish an anatomically correct elbow joint conformation. While it is generally agreed that a fractured coronoid process should be removed, it is controversial whether a fractured anconeal process should be removed or re-attached during the procedure (Schwarz and Shires 2004 b; Brunnberg, Burger et al. 2005).

3.9.1.5 Prognosis

Prognosis for OCD surgery depends on the affected joint(s). It is good to excellent for the shoulder joint, and fair to guarded for the elbow, stifle and hock joint. In these latter joints, it is probable that DJD will eventually ensue despite surgical treatment (Schwarz and Shires 2004 a).

Prognosis for elbow dysplasia is fair to good with surgical treatment, although the eventual development of DJD is to be expected (Schwarz and Shires 2004 b).

3.9.2 Epizootology

Few numbers concerning incidence and prevalence of OC(D) in Irish Wolfhounds have been published in the veterinary literature. One study found that 4 out of 45 Wolfhounds (8.9%) in a clinical database were affected (Necas, Dvorak et al. 1999). Another study found that their relative risk as compared to all dog breeds seems to be about 3.5 times higher (see chapter 3.14.1). The OFA database lists 272 screened Irish Wolfhounds, of which 11.8% had abnormal elbows (Anonymous 2005 b).

3.9.3 Heredity and Control Measures

The diseases within the OC/OCD/ED spectrum are inherited on a polygenic base in combination with environmental interaction, with heritability values varying from 0.25 to 0.45. Due to this high heritability, it is recommended not to breed affected animals and not to repeat matings that have produced affected individuals (Schwarz and Shires 2004 a; Schwarz and Shires 2004 b). As with all polygenic diseases, the use of estimated breeding values (EBVs) would be the means of choice to reduce their incidence in a population (van Hagen, Janss et al. 2004).

To reduce the environmentally mediated risk component of disease development, it has been suggested to reduce both caloric and protein intake in growing dogs (Schawalder 1997). However, there is a certain risk that this measure may conceal an existing genetic predisposition and thus be detrimental to selection.

3.10 Von Willebrand's Disease (vWD)

3.10.1 Description

Von Willebrand's Disease is the most common inherited disorder of haemostasis in the domestic dog and has been described in at least 60 breeds. There have been reports on its occurrence in Irish Wolfhounds (Clark and Parry 1995).

3.10.1.1 Pathophysiology

Von Willebrand factor (vWf) is a large glycoprotein, which circulates in the plasma as a complex with factor VIII. It is necessary for platelet adhesion to collagen and for preventing rapid factor VIII clearance from the circulation. Various genetic defects in vWf may lead to decreased platelet function and thus delayed blood coagulation. Several types have been described, with type I leading to decreased quantities of vWf in the blood. This can cause haemorrhages into a variety of organs (Kociba and Kruth 2004).

3.10.1.2 Symptoms

The disease seems to be subclinical in Irish Wolfhounds (Clark and Parry 1995), although excessive bleeding as a result of injury or surgery is a possible complication (Kociba and Kruth 2004).

3.10.1.3 Diagnosis

A history of increased bleeding tendency should warrant mucosal bleeding time and laboratory tests. Von Willebrand Factor plasma concentrations can be measured with a commercially available ELISA – a concentration of >70 Canine Units (CU) per decilitre has been described as normal in dogs. However, a survey of 41 Wolfhounds from Australia found that only 20% of these dogs had a vWf within normal range (Clark and Parry 1995). Reference values for other breeds may thus not apply to Irish Wolfhounds.

Differential diagnoses include classic haemophilia (which has not been reported in Irish Wolfhounds), and other inherited or acquired haemostasis defects, such as warfarin poisoning.

3.10.1.4 Therapy

Given that vWD has a hereditary base, there is no curative therapy available today. Affected dogs should be closely monitored for 48 hours after surgery. A concentrated cryoprecipitate of vWf and factor VIII is available for clinically manifest vWD. Alternatively, plasma or whole blood may be given. As opposed to haemophilia VIII, the bleeding can usually be controlled with one or two transfusions (Kociba and Kruth 2004).

There have been reports that subclinical hypothyreosis may increase the bleeding tendency in vWD. Thyroxin supplementation may thus be an alternative treatment option in such cases (Kociba and Kruth 2004).

3.10.1.5 Prognosis

The clinical course and prognosis depend on the plasma concentration of vWf. Since no relationship between vWf concentrations and bleeding tendency has been established in Irish Wolfhounds, prognosis can be regarded as excellent as long as no clinical symptoms are evident (Clark and Parry 1995). Nevertheless, animals with low vWf concentrations should be closely monitored after surgery as mentioned above.

3.10.2 Epizootology

The previously mentioned study of 41 Irish Wolfhounds from Australia (Clark and Parry 1995) found that 20% of dogs had vWf values within the normal range (>70 CU/dl), 22% had equivocal values (50-70 CU/dl), and 58% had low values (<50 CU/dl). Of these with low values, 21% had values <36 CU/dl, which was shown to be a clinical threshold for increased bleeding tendency in Dobermans (Stokol, Parry et al. 1995). Nevertheless, none of the examined dogs had any history of an increased bleeding tendency.

3.10.3 Heredity and Control Measures

It is generally agreed that the breed-specific mutations that lead to a decrease in vWf production follow an intermediary mode of inheritance, with dogs with normal values having two normal alleles, dogs with equivocal values having one defective allele, and dogs with low values having two defective alleles (Kociba and Kruth 2004). Additionally, it has been suggested that in humans, this autosomal locus may control an independent locus on the X chromosome that itself controls a part of normal vWf expression (Miller, Graham et al. 1979 a; Miller, Graham et al. 1979 b).

However, no exact study of heredity has been undertaken in Irish Wolfhounds. While the low clinical relevance of vWD in the breed makes it unlikely to be a deciding factor for breeding, it would at least seem reasonable not to breed two animals with vWf plasma values under 36 CU/dl to each other and to exclude animals with clinically manifest increased bleeding tendency and concurrently low vWf from breeding.

3.11 Progressive Retinal Atrophy (PRA)

3.11.1 Description

Progressive Retinal Atrophy is a generic term for a group of genetically heterogeneous conditions that lead to degeneration of the retina and subsequent blindness (Smith and Miller 2004). Although only very little information on the occurrence of PRA in Irish Wolfhounds is available in the veterinary literature (Gould, Petersen-Jones et al. 1997), personal communications and lay articles from breeders and breed-specific charity organisations indicate that it occurs in the breed (Thornton 2005).

3.11.1.1 Pathophysiology

The molecular pathophysiology of PRA varies between breeds depending on the underlying mutation. Notably, numerous genetic defects in the photoreceptor mechanism are responsible for progressive photoreceptor degeneration (Smith and Miller 2004). The underlying mutation has not been identified in Irish Wolfhounds; therefore, the exact pathophysiology of PRA in the breed remains unknown.

3.11.1.2 Symptoms

Lay reports indicate that affected Wolfhounds seem to first show symptoms at around two to three years of age (Thornton 2005), although ophthalmoscopic changes become apparent earlier (Sargan, personal communication). Symptoms start with night blindness, which progressively affects vision in bright light until complete blindness is present. Patient history may mimic acute blindness when blind animals are introduced into unfamiliar surroundings. The disease process is painless (Smith and Miller 2004).

3.11.1.3 Diagnosis

In affected animals, direct and consensual pupillary reflexes are impaired or absent. During ophthalmoscopic examination, tapetal hyperreflectivity and/or nontapetal depigmentation as well as retinal blood vessel attenuation and optic nerve atrophy may be found. Both eyes are affected symmetrically.

Concerning differential diagnosis, PRA can be differentiated from other possible causes of slowly progressive vision loss, such as cataracts, retinal scarring, pigmentation or oedema, posterior uveitis etc. by ophthalmoscopy. Experimentally, severe vitamin A and E deficiency has been shown to cause retinal degeneration in dogs (Smith and Miller 2004).

3.11.1.4 Therapy

The disease is currently incurable and its progress unstoppable. Blind dogs should be kept in a familiar environment and only walked on a leash. Practical suggestions to improve quality of life include avoiding to change the position of furniture, using dog toys that produce sound, and applying perfume to the pieces of furniture to help the dogs identify their position (Smith and Miller 2004).

3.11.1.5 Prognosis

Affected animals will gradually and irreversibly turn completely blind. Nevertheless, properly managed dogs have a normal life expectancy, unless they have to be euthanised due to an inability to adapt to blindness.

3.11.2 Epizootology

Very little information on incidence and prevalence of PRA in the Wolfhound population is available. It seems that only 4 new cases were registered with the Irish Wolfhound Foundation during from 1997 to 2007, with roughly 4'000 Wolfhounds registered per year (Janis, personal communication). On the other hand, it is quite probable that there are additional unreported cases. Nevertheless, the incidence of PRA in Wolfhounds seems to be low at the moment.

3.11.3 Heredity and Control Measures

While a mutation in the *rom-1* structural gene has been excluded as the cause for PRA in Irish Wolfhounds (Gould, Petersen-Jones et al. 1997), the exact molecular genetic base of the disease in the breed remains unknown. A simple autosomal recessive mode of inheritance has been postulated; recommended control measures are thus not to breed known carriers (parents of affected offspring) and full siblings of affected dogs (2/3 risk of being a carrier). A lay article available on the internet includes a list of carriers identified through their production of affected offspring (Thornton 2005).

3.12 Miscellaneous

3.12.1 Odds Ratios for different diseases

Dorn (2002) has published Odds Ratio comparisons for dogs of 78 breeds for which more than 1'000 cases were available in the Veterinary Medical Database of Purdue University, using the 10 most frequently diagnosed diseases in the respective breeds. He investigated whether the disease risk of the specific breeds in question differed significantly from the risk for the average population in the database. His findings for Irish Wolfhounds are quoted in table 3.7 (Odds Ratio for diseases of average frequency would equal 1. P values were calculated using Pearson's Chi-square test).

Disease	N° of Cases	Odds Ratio	95 % CI	P value
Cancer (OS)	80	27.50	21.21 – 35.66	<0.01
Bloat	86	5.52	4.38 – 6.95	<0.01
OCD	62	3.65	2.80 – 4.75	<0.01
Heart Disease	251	3.43	2.93 – 4.01	<0.01
Urinary Disease	34	1.37	0.97 – 1.94	>0.05 / **NS**
Lame, weak limb	52	0.85	0.64 – 1.13	>0.05 / **NS**
Diarrhoea	38	0.69	0.50 – 0.96	<0.05
Hypothyroidism	30	0.36	0.25 – 0.52	<0.01
Dermal disease	32	0.30	0.21 – 0.42	<0.01
Hip Dysplasia	33	0.09	0.06 – 0.13	<0.01

Table 3.7: Odds Ratios for the ten most commonly diagnosed diseases in Irish Wolfhounds in the Veterinary Medical Database as compared to the overall dog population (Dorn 2002). OS = Osteosarcoma; OCD = Osteochondritis dissecans; CI = Confidence Interval; NS = Not Significant

It is interesting to note that even though hypothyroidism is sometimes mentioned as a breed-specific problem in Irish Wolfhounds, the Odds Ratio publication in this study shows that the breed has a considerably lower risk of being affected with the disease as compared to the overall dog population. The low incidence of hip dysplasia may also be surprising in a giant breed, but can probably be explained by the sighthound-like hip anatomy of the breed, where the comparably steep pelvic angle leads to an improved pressure distribution of the femoral head on the hip socket due to an increase of the pressure area.

3.12.2 Below-Average Male Fertility

Poor male fertility parameters (low libido, decreased sperm quality and testicular softening) have been described to occur more commonly in Irish Wolfhounds than they do in the overall dog population, and to progress more rapidly as the dogs age. The reasons for this are unclear, but serum testosterone levels did not vary significantly between a sample of male Irish Wolfhounds and the control population (Dahlbom, Andersson et al. 1995; Dahlbom, Andersson et al. 1997).

3.12.3 Calcinosis Circumscripta

Calcinosis circumscripta (calcium gout) was described in the tongue of a 10-month-old male Irish Wolfhound (Douglas and Kelly 1966). Additionally, two cases of the disease were described on the toes of 3-year-old Irish Wolfhound bitch (in whose case swelling had first been noted at 1 year of age) and her 10-month-old daughter. The sire as well as the only sibling of the latter bitch did not show clinical abnormalities (Owen 1967).

3.12.4 Extraocular Myositis and Acquired Strabismus

Strabismus following conjunctivitis was reported in four related Irish Wolfhounds (Wolfer 1995). A later study described three cases where strabismus developed as a result of extraocular myositis and subsequent fibrosis (Allgoewer, Blair et al. 2000). The three animals in the latter study had already been described by Wolfer (1995) (Wolfer, personal communication) – the total number of cases in the literature is thus four Irish Wolfhounds

Successful therapy consisted of surgical resection of the inflamed/contracted muscle in combination with immunosuppression. Given the relatedness of the animals in these studies, a hereditary component is possible.

3.12.5 Cervical Spondylomyelopathy (Wobbler Syndrome)

Cervical spondylomyelopathy has been reported to occur in Irish Wolfhounds. The intervertebral space of C3-C4 seems to be most frequently affected in the breed. The aetiology of the condition is uncertain, although genetic predisposition, over-nutrition and osteochondrosis (see chapter 3.9) have been suggested to play a role in its development. Signs are most commonly observed before the end of skeletal maturation, although they may also become evident at a later age (Ettinger and Feldman 1995).

The disease is clinically characterised by the effects of chronic compression of the spinal marrow in the cervical region. Notably, increased hind limb spinal reflexes (upper motor neuron) can be observed. Diagnosis should be made through radiography and myelography to demonstrate the presence of a dynamic cervical compression. The potential risks and benefits of stress myelography as a means of diagnosis are discussed controversially (Ettinger and Feldman 1995).

3.12.6 Cataracts

There is one report on the occurrence of hereditary cataracts in Irish Wolfhounds (Krohne 2001). Two types can be discerned, which are divided by the dogs' age at onset: young dogs become affected at age 1 to 2, while older dogs become affected at age 5 to 7. The cataract is located in the posterior cortical region and seldom impairs vision. The CERF recommends not to breed affected individuals and to examine their relatives for the presence of the condition. No published data on incidence and prevalence of the condition are available, and a later study on the subject does not mention Irish Wolfhounds (Gelatt and Mackay 2005).

3.12.7 Atypical Hepatic Encephalopathy

The occurrence of an atypical hepatic encephalopathy as a probable consequence of PSS was described in two Irish Wolfhound siblings in 2003. As opposed to what is generally seen in hepatic encephalopathy, the white matter was not predominantly involved. Histologically, widespread spongiform changes in the neuropil, fibre bundles interspersed within the grey matter and some neuronal vacuoles could be observed. No infectious agents (rabies or distemper virus, prion proteins) were detected (Herden, Beineke et al. 2003).

3.12.8 Spinal Nephroblastoma

A spinal nephroblastoma was described in a yearling Irish Wolfhound male from South Africa, leading to slowly progressive paresis of the left hind limb (Vaughan-Scott, Goldin et al. 1999). This intradural, extramedullary tumour has been described under various names (e.g. neuroepithelioma, hamartoma, ependymoma, medulloepithelioma), occurring infrequently between T10 and L2 in young large breed dogs. In the dog in question, it was diagnosed through myelography and cerebrospinal fluid analysis, which showed an intradural, extramedullary mass and the presence of neoplastic cells respectively. Diagnosis was confirmed post mortem through histopathology.

Given that as opposed to the reported case, clinical symptom onset is usually described as sudden, this tumour type should be taken into consideration as a differential diagnosis for FCE (see chapter 3.7.1). Prognosis for complete recovery after surgical excision is guarded to poor; the dog in the study was euthanised during surgery due to infiltrative tumour growth.

3.12.9 Juvenile Nephropathy

Juvenile nephropathy (defined as renal disease in an immature animal that is not related to primary renal inflammatory processes) was described in a 7-month-old male Irish Wolfhound in 2000. The clinical signs included anorexia, exercise intolerance, ulcerative gingivitis, polyuria and polydipsia, and an episode of haematemesis and melena. Radiographically, kidneys were small, with irregular margins. Gross necropsy showed a large number of small cysts (1 mm in diameter) in the cortex, as well as multiple acute gastric ulceration (Peeters, Clercx et al. 2000).

Microscopically, extensive connective tissue deposits were observed, within which dilated tubuli as well as abnormal glomeruli could be seen. Glomeruli showed cystic dilation of the urinary space, but immature glomeruli were not observed. Some of the tubuli were lined by hyperchromatic tall-cubuoidal epithelium. Also, mild, focal mononuclear inflammation was observed.

In the authors' conclusion, these findings imply that the metanephric blastema failed to undergo complete differentiation. Given that nephrogenesis is incomplete at birth in dogs, the disease could have a hereditary base, but postnatal or fetal insults are also possible aetiological explanations. Nevertheless, since hereditary juvenile nephropathies have been described in various dog breeds, it is advised that relatives of an affected dog should be screened for the disease to avoid its possible spread.

3.12.10 Cricopharyngeal Achalasia

A case of dysphagia caused by cricopharyngeal achalasia was described in a 5-month-old Irish Wolfhound bitch (Niles, Williams et al. 2001). This rare congenital disease often leads to secondary aspiration pneumonia. Treatment was surgical through lateral cricopharyngeal myectomy and resulted in rapid recovery.

The authors describe fluoroscopic evaluation of swallowing using barium as contrast medium and conclude that cricopharyngeal achalasia should be included in the differential diagnosis of swallowing disorders in young dogs. Other differential diagnoses include foreign bodies, megaoesophagus, space-occupying lesions, strictures, and trauma-induced lesions.

3.12.11 Large Granular Intestinal Lymphosarcoma

A five-year-old spayed Irish Wolfhound bitch was diagnosed with a large granular lymphocyte (LGL) tumour which diffusely invaded the intestinal walls, leading to gastrointestinal symptoms and weight loss that did not react to the usual therapeutic approaches. Apart from a slight thrombocytopenia, blood cell count was normal; however, abnormal granular lymphocytes could be identified in a blood smear after the diagnosis had been made through endoscopy and histopathology. No lymphadenopathies were evident at the time of diagnosis. The bitch was euthanised upon diagnosis due to the poor prognosis of the disease.

LGL are very rare in dogs and are thought to mainly arise from T-cells, with a minority arising from Natural Killer (NK) cells. While the aetiology of the disease is unknown, a viral component may play a role in its development. A possible hereditary component has not been investigated. Differential diagnoses include lymphocytosis due to an increased number of reactive T-cells, which can for example be seen in *Ehrlichia canis* infections (Snead 2007).

3.12.12 Paediatric *Neospora caninum* Myositis

A seven-week old female Irish Wolfhound puppy was presented with abnormal hind limb gait, which had first been seen at four weeks of age and had been treated as "Swimmer Syndrome". The dog was alert, but had abnormal hind limb positioning (excessive abduction and outward rotation) and walked with both stifles flexed. Both quadriceps muscles were atrophied, and patellar reflexes were absent on both sides. Proprioception was normal, however (Crookshanks, Taylor et al. 2007).

Diagnostic procedures included radiography, myelography, electromyography, and muscle and nerve biopsies. Serum titers against *Toxoplasma gondii* and *Neospora caninum* were also measured. These showed a strongly increased IgG titer for *Neospora*. The dam and one of the tested littermates were also seropositive for the organism, but did not show clinical signs. Immunostaining of muscle biopsies showed disseminated clusters of *N. caninum*, resulting in myositis. Treatment included clindamycin and physiotherapy, which resulted in marked improvement within four weeks. Treatment was continued for 18 weeks in total, resulting in an almost complete remission. The bitch had a normal life and was euthanised at age nine due to an unrelated condition.

3.12.13 Pure White Cell Aplasia

A three-year-old Irish Wolfhound was presented with acute fever and lethargy. Blood cell count showed the complete absence of neutrophiles, which could be shown to be due to granulocyte aplasia in the bone marrow. Laboratory work was consistent with the presence of anti-neutrophile antibodies, indicating an autoimmune disease process. The dog was treated with steroidal and non-steroidal immunosuppressives, but episodes of neutropenia continued. Eventually, neutrophile count could be stabilised in the low normal range with prednisone 0.4 mg/kg p.o. once every 48 hours and azathioprine 2 mg/kg SID, which was successful for 15 months. The dog then developed multiple secondary problems such as autoimmune haemolytic anaemia and thrombocytopenia, nasal aspergillosis and septicaemia, which resulted in euthanasia on day 784 (Weiss and Henson 2007).

3.12.14 Incisor Restoration

For the sake of completeness, it should be mentioned that a technique to restore a fractured upper incisor tooth (I3) was described in an 18-month-old Irish Wolfhound. Upon re-inspection ten months after the procedure, the tooth was found to be fully functional and non-mobile (Adams and Gillespie 1979).

3.13 Clinical Reference Values

3.13.1 Growth Patterns

The growth patterns of Irish Wolfhounds were studied and compared to three other large breeds: the Newfoundland, Leonberger and Labrador Retriever (Trangerud, Grondalen et al. 2007). Growth was measured in these four breeds through body weight (BW) and compared to alkaline phosphatise activity (ALP) and the circumference of the distal radius and ulna (CDRU). The study included a total of 700 dogs derived from 107 litters born in Norway between November 1998 and June 2001. 99 of these dogs were Irish Wolfhounds; at the time of analysis, 81 were still part of the study. Results for the breed are provided in table 3.10.

Parameter	Males	Females
Birth weight (g)	631.00 ± 14.1	582.00 ± 11.4
Mature weight (kg)	65.71 ± 0.40	55.34 ± 0.39
Age at peak growth (days)	104.60 ± 1.03	94.67 ± 1.02
Age at end of growth (days)	405.30 ± 5.75	367.40 ± 5.76

Table 3.10: Growth parameters as measured in a population of Irish Wolfhounds from Norway (Trangerud, Grondalen et al. 2007). All variabilities are given as Standard Errors as used in the study.

CDRU peaked at around 180 days of age, then declined and stabilised at around one year of age. Males had a significantly higher circumference than females at all ages. Breed differences in ALP levels were strongest at age 90 days and then gradually diminished, until there was no measurable breed difference in adult dogs. This is explained by the fact that ALP is an indicator of bone turnover, which is increased proportionally to the speed of growth of a given breed.

3.13.2 General Haematology

Clark and Parry (1997) published reference values for general haematology based on n=22 clinically healthy Irish Wolfhounds from Australia, which are reproduced below:

Value	Mean ± SD	Total Range
PCV	0.49 ± 0.04	0.40 - 0.57
Red Cell Count (*10^{12}/L)	6.80 ± 0.60	5.70 - 8.10
Haemoglobin (g/L)	17.40 ± 1.50	14.40 - 20.40
MCV (fL)	66.80 ± 1.80	64.00 - 70.00
MCH (pg)	25.50 ± 1.00	24.00 - 27.00
MCHC (g/L)	38.30 ± 0.60	37.00 - 40.00
Leukocyte count (*10^9/L)	8.40 ± 1.50	5.30 - 11.60
Bands (%)	1.30 ± 1.10	N/A
Neutrophiles (%)	63.30 ± 9.40	N/A
Lymphocytes (%)	20.10 ± 7.20	N/A
Monocytes (%)	8.60 ± 3.40	N/A
Eosinophiles (%)	6.70 ± 4.30	N/A
Bands (*10^9/L)	0.10 ± 0.09	0.00 - 0.30
Neutrophiles (*10^9/L)	5.30 ± 0.80	3.70 - 6.90
Lymphocytes (*10^9/L)	1.70 ± 0.10	1.50 - 1.90
Monocytes (*10^9/L)	0.70 ± 0.06	0.30 - 1.60
Eosinophiles (*10^9/L)	0.60 ± 0.05	0.40 - 0.80
Platelets (*10^9/L)	196.00 ± 48.0	110.00 - 280.00
Total plasma solids (g/L)	67.10 ± 2.60	61.00 - 73.00

Table 3.8: Haematology values of 22 clinically healthy Irish Wolfhounds from Australia (Clark and Parry 1997). SD = Standard Deviation, PCV = Packed Cell Volume, MCV = Mean Corpuscular Volume, MCH = Mean Corpuscular Haemoglobin, MCHC = Mean Corpuscular Haemoglobin Content

The population on which these values are based consisted of 8 males and 14 females from 16 months to 9 years of age. No significant gender differences were found.

It is interesting to notice that even though they are usually considered sighthounds, Irish Wolfhounds in this study had values similar to non-sighthound breeds rather than Greyhounds, which are routinely used as a reference for all sighthound breeds. The only significant difference was the platelet count, which was lower than the values found in non-sighthounds, but higher than the values reported in Greyhounds. The authors suggest thus that Greyhound reference values should not be used for Irish Wolfhound blood. However, it should also be pointed out that the relatively low number of dogs as well as the geographic isolation of the population might have had an effect on these results.

3.13.3 Blood Pressure

Blood pressure reference values were established in n=158 non-sedated Irish Wolfhounds of normal body condition score that had passed a clinical cardiovascular examination and an electrocardiogram and whose clinical history as given by the owner did not indicate any signs of cardiovascular disease (Bright and Dentino 2002). Measures were taken repeatedly at the coccygeal artery, using the oscillometric technique. Mean systolic pressure was found to be 116.0 mm Hg, mean diastolic pressure was 69.2 mm HG, and mean arterial pressure was 87.8 mm Hg. There was no significant difference in systolic blood pressure between standing and recumbent Wolfhounds, but diastolic pressure was slightly, yet significantly lower in standing animals as compared to animals in lateral recumbency.

A highly significant effect (P<0.0001) of age on blood pressure values was found in mature animals (>24 months old), with older animals having a tendency to have increased blood pressure within this cohort. However, no such correlation was found in animals <24 months of age. Furthermore, significant differences in values existed between dogs that were considered calm vs. anxious at the time of examination. Anxiousness was assessed by the same person during the whole study, with criteria including trembling, flinching, and requiring manual restraint. A summary of the results is given in table 3.9.

Cohort	n	Systolic AP	Diastolic AP	Mean AP	Heart Rate
<24 months	65	111.0 (1.4)	65.3 (1.2)	84.2 (1.2)	112.4 (1.8)
>24 months	88	122.8 (1.3)	74.0 (1.0)	93.5 (1.1)	112.6 (1.6)
Calm	75	113.8 (1.42)	68.2 (1.0)	86.5 (1.0)	109.6 (1.5)
Anxious	67	120.0 (1.5)	71.1 (1.2)	91.2 (1.3)	115.6 (1.9)
All dogs	158	116.0 (1.4)	69.2 (1.2)	87.8 (1.2)	112.5 (1.5)

Table 3.9: Blood pressure measurements and Standard Error (in parentheses) in different cohorts of healthy Irish Wolfhounds (Bright and Dentino 2002). AP = arterial blood pressure. Blood pressure measurements are indicated in mm Hg. Mood was not assessed in the initial 16 evaluated dogs.

The finding that anxious animals exhibited an increased blood pressure is not particularly surprising and reproduces findings from a previous study, in which temperament was found do be a good predictor for blood pressure in dogs (Vincent and Michell 1996). The tendency of an increase in blood pressure in older animals mirrors the tendency to have an increased blood pressure in older humans and also reproduces previous findings in dogs (Bodey and Michell 1996).

There is little research concerning high blood pressure as a risk factor in dogs. A more recent study describes a link between obesity and high blood pressure in the dog (Montoya, Morris et al. 2006), which would presumably also apply to Irish Wolfhounds.

4 Dogs, Materials and Methods

4.1 Dogs

Pedigree data were collected from various national studbooks, specialised publications (Graham 1906/1959; Murphy 1991), and club yearbooks (Anonymous 1922-2005). Further data were taken from breeders' records, personal communications from veterinary researchers and the electronic databases of both Small Animal Clinics of the Vetsuisse Faculty in Berne and Zurich. At the time of analysis, the pedigree database contained n=50'822 individuals born between 1862 and 2005. Lifespan data were known for n=2016 individuals, while causes of death were known for n=530 individuals. The whole of these data are summarised as "present data" and analysed in chapter 6.

Additionally, information on lifespan and causes of death of n=572 and n=161 individuals respectively was obtained from two previously published North American studies (Bernardi 1986; Prokopenko 1998), the data of which were provided by their respective authors for re-analysis. The data were anonymised, i.e. no pedigree information was available for the dogs in them.

Information on lifespan of n=627 UK/Irish dogs and data of n=838 dogs alive by the end of the year 1990 were also available (Murphy 1991). As opposed to the two other databases, these included detailed pedigree information. Due to statistical considerations (significant differences between databases; differing threshold definitions of right censored data), all three of these databases were analysed separately from the data in our main database (see chapter 5).

4.2 Software

4.2.1 Pedigree Explorer (PedX)

Pedigree Explorer® (de Jong 2002-2006) is a commercially available software (www.breedmate.com) that allows the displaying of pedigrees, pedigree charts, reverse pedigrees etc. and calculates Wright's Inbreeding Coefficients (COI) and Coefficients of Relationship (COR) over any desired number of generations. The program has a "Data Doc" function that checks for the presence of double entries by name and/or registration number and can also find and correct similarly written names, individuals born before their parents, self-parenting errors etc. The program is compatible with Microsoft Excel® as well as Microsoft Access®.

In this study, Pedigree Explorer version 5.4.1 was used for data storage and management, the search for and correction of double entries and similar names and the calculation of Wright's Inbreeding Coefficients over 5, 10 and 20 generations.

4.2.2 The SAS Program Package

Statistical analyses were performed in The SAS System® Version 8.02. Graphs were created using The SAS System (boxplots) and Microsoft Excel (all other graphs). A probability level of $p \leq 0.05$ was considered statistically significant.

Statistical tests used included chi-square and Fisher's exact test for categorical distributions (PROC FREQ). Analyses of variance as well as regression analyses were performed with PROC GLM.

The SAS System was also used for data management, notably for converting the Microsoft Excel Spreadsheets derived from PedX into a form that the PEDIG applications were able to read.

4.2.3 PEDIG

PEDIG is a freely available FORTRAN program package that can be used for the analysis of large amounts of pedigree data (Heuch and Li 1972). In this study, Meuwissen's Inbreeding Coefficients were calculated using the "meuw.exe" program of the PEDIG package, while the calculations of ancestor analyses (probabilities of gene origins) were performed using the "prob_orig.exe" program.

The prob_orig.exe program computes the probabilities of gene origin for a user-defined population of individuals over a user-defined number of generations. These probabilities are combined all together to estimate an effective number of founders. The program then calculates the non-zero contributions of each founder to the studied population.

prob_orig.exe was used to study the differences in contribution of different founders to populations of dogs known to have suffered from a certain disease and dogs in a reference population. If these diseases are hereditary, it can be expected that marked founder differences between the affected and reference populations should result from this approach.

To define a reference population for animals suffering from a certain disease, 20 animals of identical year of birth and country of origin per affected case were randomly selected from the overall database. Affected animals were excluded from the sampling data. Random selection of individuals was achieved by using random numbers generated by the RANDOM procedure in Microsoft Excel.

The calculations with prob_orig.exe were executed under the assumption that there was only one gender (unisex). After the calculations, the correct genders were reassigned to the identified important ancestors for evaluation.

4.3 Definition of Causes of Death

When available, causes of death were divided into eight categories as specified in table 4.1. Reservations concerning classification bias (chapter 3.1.1.2) particularly apply to category 2:

Nr	Cause	Nr	Cause
1	Gastric Dilation Volvulus (GDV)	5	Infectious/Inflammatory (II)
2	Dilatative Cardiomyopathy (DCM)	6	Accidental Death (Acc)
3	Osteogenic Sarcoma (OS)	7	Other General Debilitation (OGD)
4	Other Cancer (OCa)	8	Unknown Reason

Table 4.1: Classification of causes of death in this study

Category number 7, "Other General Debilitation", was defined as a known cause of death that did not occur frequently enough to warrant a separate category, but did not qualify as "Unknown" either. This includes, amongst other causes, renal and hepatic failure, intestinal volvulus, epileptic seizures, degenerative joint disease etc.

4.4 Definition of Right Censored Data

Lifespan data are considered to be right censored whenever individuals that were born before the end of a data collection period are still alive at the end of the said period. This phenomenon will cause an artificial decrease in the measured lifespan due to the fact that death data of these individuals will not be included (also see chapter 3.1.1.3). Given the association of this phenomenon with the birth cohorts studied, it was decided to call it "Cohort Bias" in this study (Urfer 2008).

In order to arrive at a representative lifespan estimate, right censored data must be corrected before analysis. In our case, this was achieved by excluding all individuals born less than twelve years before the end of data collection from our data. This time duration was reached through the fact that only extremely few dogs in all available datasets had lifespans longer than these twelve years.

Given that the individual data collection periods for the databases studied ended at varying points in time, definitions of right censored data due to Cohort Bias had to be established individually for each one of them. These are provided in table 4.2. Death data of dogs born after the end of the specified year of birth were presumed to be subject to Cohort Bias in the analyses and thus excluded from analysis.

Population	Year
Bernardi	1975
Murphy	1977
Prokopenko	1986
Present Data	1993

Table 4.2: Definitions of right censored data (Cohort Bias) by population

5 Results of Past Studies Revisited

5.1 Re-analysis of Bernardi (1986) and Prokopenko (1998)

5.1.1 Data Merging

As discussed in chapters 3.1.3.1 and 3.1.3.3, the original data of Bernardi (1986) were available to us, consisting of n=582 individuals in anonymised form. Also available were the original data of Prokopenko (1998), consisting of n=161 individuals in partially anonymised form. When adjusted for Cohort Bias, n=327 individuals from Bernardi (1986) and n=72 individuals from Prokopenko (1998) remained. Causes of death were classified as discussed in chapter 4.3

ANOVA showed that lifespan data (P=0.75), distribution of causes of death (P=0.99), sex (P=0.91) and castration frequency (P=0.37) were not significantly different in both populations. A General Linear Model analysis for these four variables analysed by population resulted in a P=0.86 and no significant single variable effects/interactions. Therefore, the data from both studies were merged into one database for analysis.

5.1.2 Population Structure

The database consisted of n=399 dogs, 186 males (173 intact/13 castrated) and 213 females (138/75), born between 1954 and 1986. Gender distribution was not significantly different from an equal distribution model (P=0.18, chi-square=1.82). Significantly more females than males had been castrated (P<0.0001; chi-square=46.00). Birth cohorts were distributed as reproduced in figure 5.1 below.

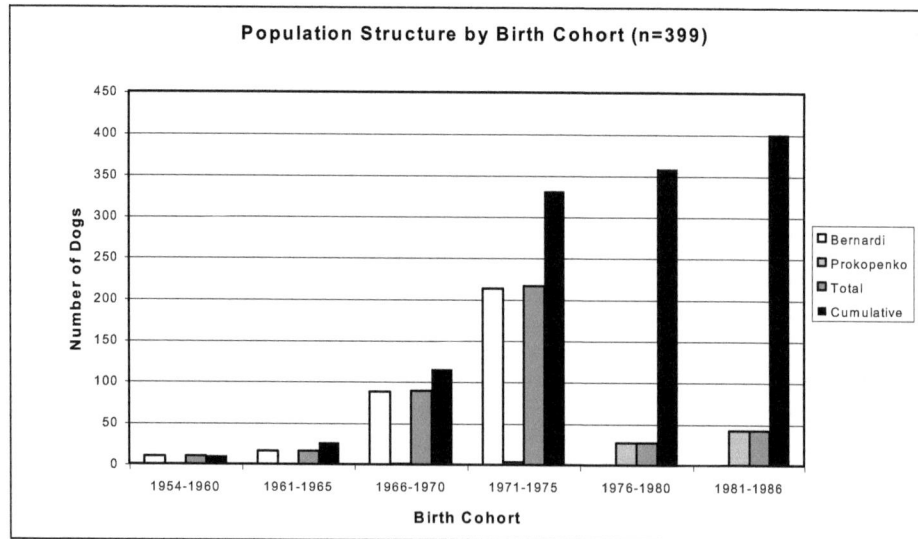

Fig. 5.1: Population structure of Bernardi (1986) and Prokopenko (1998), adjusted for Cohort Bias

5.1.3 Lifespan and Survival

It is unclear whether the lifespans of these dogs are normally distributed (Shapiro-Wilk P=0.0014; Kolmogorov-Smirnov P=0.067). Given the borderline nature of these results, it was decided to work with a non-normal distribution model. Statistical measures are given in Table 5.1:

Measure	Value (years)
Mean age ± SD	7.35 ± 2.64
Minimum	0.33
5% of dogs dead	2.33
1st quartile	5.75
Median age	7.50
3rd quartile	9.34
95% of dogs dead	11.50
Maximum	13.50

Table 5.1: Lifespan distributions in the merged Bernardi/Prokopenko data; adjusted for Cohort Bias.

The overall survival curve at birth is given in figure 5.2 below:

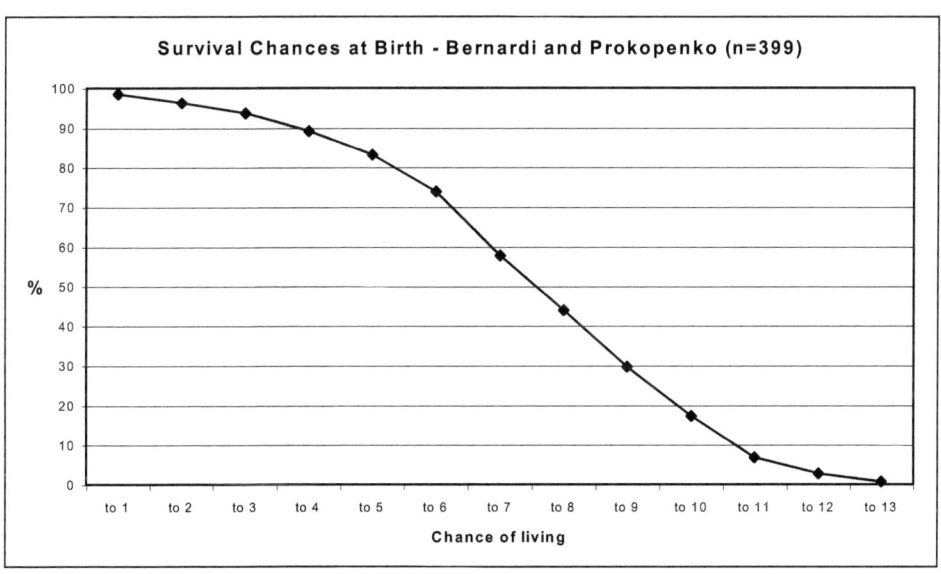

Fig. 5.2: Overall survival curve for the Bernardi/Prokopenko data; adjusted for Cohort Bias.

5.1.4 Causes of Death

5.1.4.1 Influence of Cohort Bias

The distribution of causes of death was analysed within the dogs removed during Cohort Bias adjustment (n=340) and the adjusted population (n=399) was compared. Results were borderline for the overall population (P=0.076, Mantel-Haenszel chi-square=3.15) and significant or almost significant for several disease classes (DCM: P=0.054, Fisher's left-sided test; P=0.087, chi-square=2.93; P=0.096, Fisher's two-sided test. Accidents: P=0.03, chi-square=4.70. Unknown causes: P=0.0004, chi-square=12.52). It was therefore decided to use only the adjusted population for analysis.

5.1.4.2 Adjusted for Cohort Bias

When the dogs that were subject to Cohort Bias were excluded, Causes of Death were distributed as shown in table 5.2:

Cause of Death	n	%	Mean age ± SD
GDV	47	11.78	6.54 ± 2.15
DCM	67	16.79	7.92 ± 2.14
OS	79	19.80	6.88 ± 2.03
OCa	48	12.03	7.39 ± 2.34
II	22	5.51	6.56 ± 2.89
Accident	21	5.26	5.82 ± 3.92
OGD	67	16.79	7.64 ± 3.25
Unknown	48	12.03	8.66 ± 2.38

Table 5.2: Mean ages at and percentual importance of different causes of death

Using a general linear model with type III SS, the effects of causes of death on lifespan were highly significant as expected. When "unknown" was considered a normal class, this resulted in P<0.0001, R^2=0.08, F=4.84, DF=7. When it was excluded, the result was P=0.0048, R^2=0.053, F=3.18, DF=6.

5.1.5 Gender and Castration Effects

5.1.5.1 Lifespan

As shown in table 5.3, female Irish Wolfhounds lived significantly longer than males (P=0.026, R^2=0.012, F=4.97, DF=1). Castration did significantly increase life expectancy over both genders (P=0.023, R^2=0.015, F=5.22, DF=1). When the population was analysed by gender, however, this effect was significant in females only, where castration resulted in a significant increase in life expectancy as compared to both intact females (P=0.039, R^2=0.023, F=4.35, DF=1) and the overall population (P=0.0045, R^2=0.023, F=8.18, DF=1). Although life expectancy was decreased in castrated males, this effect was not significant when compared to both intact males (P=0.50, R^2=0.003, F=0.46, DF=1) and the overall population (P=0.41, R^2=0.002, F=0.69, DF=1). Type III SS was used for all these analyses.

	Overall	Intact	Castrated
Males	7.03 ± 2.53 years	7.07 ± 2.52 years	6.57 ± 2.79 years
Females	7.62 ± 2.70 years	7.37 ± 2.85 years	8.07 ± 2.35 years
Overall	7.35 ± 2.64 years	7.20 ± 2.67 years	7.85 ± 2.46 years

Table 5.3: Gender and castration effects on the average life expectancy ± Standard Deviation (SD) of Irish Wolfhounds. Significant effects are discussed in the text.

5.1.5.2 Causes of Death

Males were found to be at an increased risk for death by DCM (21.0% of male deaths as opposed to 13.2% of female deaths; P=0.037, χ^2=4.35; P=0.044, Fisher's two-sided test). Females were found to be at an increased risk for death by cancer other than osteogenic sarcoma (7.53% of male deaths as opposed to 16.0% of female deaths; P=0.013, Fisher's two-sided test; χ^2 not applicable). No significant gender effects were found for the other disease classes.

Based on the results published by Priester and McKay (1980), Ru, Terracini et al. (1998) and Cooley, Beranek et al. (2002), it was decided to additionally test the influence of castration on osteogenic sarcoma risk. As a result, castrated male Irish Wolfhounds were found to be at a significantly increased risk for OS as compared to the overall population: 46.15% of castrated males died of OS as opposed to 18.91% of the rest of the population (P=0.027; Fisher's two-sided test). These significance levels became borderline when compared within males only (P=0.046, Fischer's right-sided test; P=0.077, Fischer's two-sided test). As opposed to Cooley, Beranek et al. (2002), no significant effects of female castration on osteosarcoma risk were found in our overall Irish Wolfhound population (P=0.22, χ^2=1.53; P=0.26, Fischer's two-sided test) and within females only (P=0.44, χ^2=0.59; P=0.57, Fischer's two-sided test).

5.1.5.3 Generalised Linear Models

Following the calculations above, it was decided to analyse the effects of both gender and causes of death on lifespan in a Generalised Linear Model (GLM) type III SS, with unknown causes of death being either excluded or considered a separate category. The results are shown in table 5.4 below:

	Unknown Causes Excluded			Unknown Causes Included		
n in Model	350			398		
R-square	0.072			0.097		
	DF	p	F	DF	p	F
Model	7	0.0006	3.80	8	<0.0001	5.18
Cause of Death	6	0.0016	3.65	7	<0.0001	5.16
Gender	1	0.0078	7.17	1	0.0083	7.04

Table 5.4: Generalised Linear Models for the data. DF=Degrees of Freedom;

In both cases, no significant effects of castration on lifespan (over both genders) were found when using the Generalised Linear Model.

5.2 Analysis of Murphy (1991)

ANOVA showed that lifespan data provided by Murphy (1991) differed significantly from Bernardi (1986) and Prokopenko (1998) ($P<0.0001$; $F=59.05$). Murphy's work was based on British and Irish dogs, while both Bernardi's and Prokopenko's research was focused on North American dogs. Furthermore, no information on castration status and causes of death was available, but dogs were non-anonymous, allowing for the calculation of genetic parameters. The Murphy data were therefore analysed separately.

5.2.1 Death Data

5.2.1.1 Population Structure

The raw data published by Murphy (1991) consist of a pedigree database of n=4813 Irish Wolfhounds, of which 609 have information on age at death. Also included in these data was lifespan information of n=18 dogs that appeared in the pedigree section, but for which no lifespan was given by Murphy. These were extracted from an independent publication (Somerfield 1998). The total number of individuals with known lifespan is thus n=627. Adjusted for Cohort Bias, n=336 individuals (110 males / 222 females / 4 unknown) were left for analysis. The data contained significantly fewer males than females ($P<0.0001$, chi-square=37.78). Their distribution by birth cohort is rendered in figure 5.3 below.

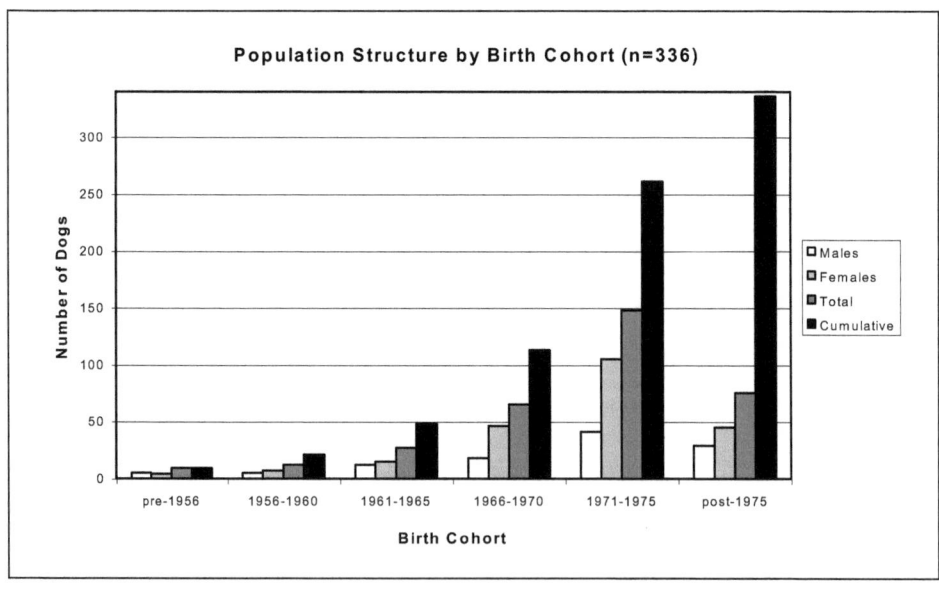

Fig. 5.3: Murphy data by birth cohort.

5.2.1.2 Lifespan and Survival

The lifespans of these dogs are not normally distributed (Shapiro-Wilk P<0.0001; Kolmogorov-Smirnov P=0.01). Statistical measures are given in Table 5.5 below:

Measure	Value (years)
Mean age ± SD	8.75 ± 2.25
Minimum	0.50
5% of dogs dead	5.00
1st quartile	7.00
Median age	9.00
3rd quartile	10.00
95% of dogs dead	12.00
Maximum	16.50

Table 5.5: Statistical parameters of the Murphy lifespan data

The overall survival curve at birth is given in figure 5.4:

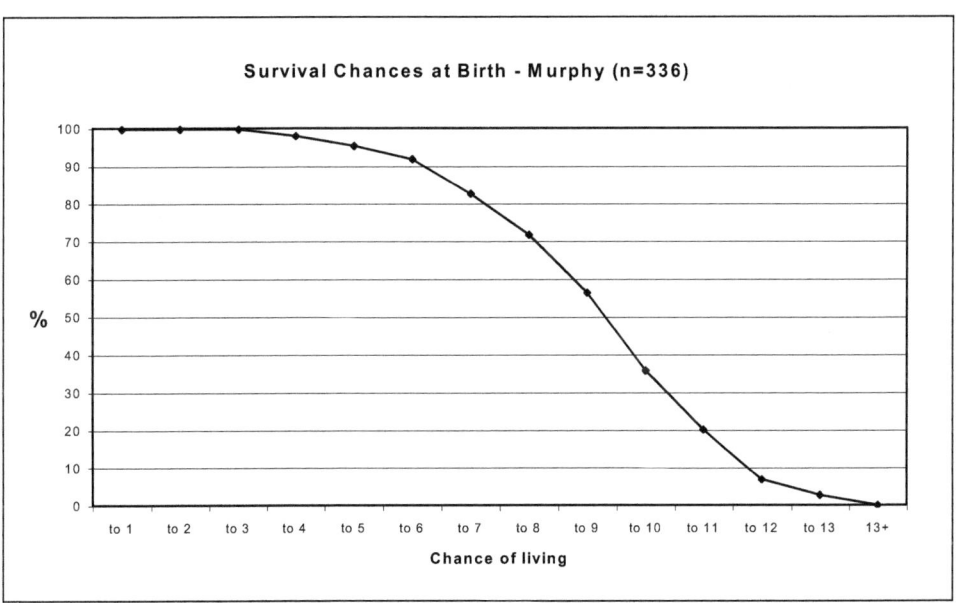

Fig. 5.4: Survival curve for the Murphy data; adjusted for Cohort Bias

5.2.1.3 Gender Effects

As mentioned already, the data contained significantly more females than males (P<0.0001 chi-square=37.78). Since no information on castration status was available, only gender effects on lifespan could be tested. However, since most of the data come from animals used for breeding purposes, the majority of individuals can be assumed to have been intact.

Group	Mean Age ± SD
All Dogs	8.75 ± 2.25 years
Males	8.33 ± 2.21 years
Females	8.94 ± 2.25 years

Table 5.6: Gender effects on lifespan in Murphy (1991)

As already observed in the Bernardi/Prokopenko data, females lived significantly longer than males in this population (P=0.022, R^2=0.016, F=5.39, DF=1; type III SS).

5.2.1.4 Inbreeding Effects

Inbreeding could be calculated in 329 Irish Wolfhounds based on the present data (see chapter 6). The possible effects of 10-generation Wright's inbreeding coefficients on measured lifespan were examined; however, no significant effects were found (P=0.82, R^2=0.00015, F=0.05, DF=1; type III SS). COIs over 5 and 20 generations as well as Meuwissen's inbreeding coefficients were also non-significant (P=0.62/R^2=0.0008/F=0.25; P=0.99/R^2=0.000001/F=0.00; P=0.32/R^2=0.003/F=0.98). The results are rendered graphically in figure 5.5 below:

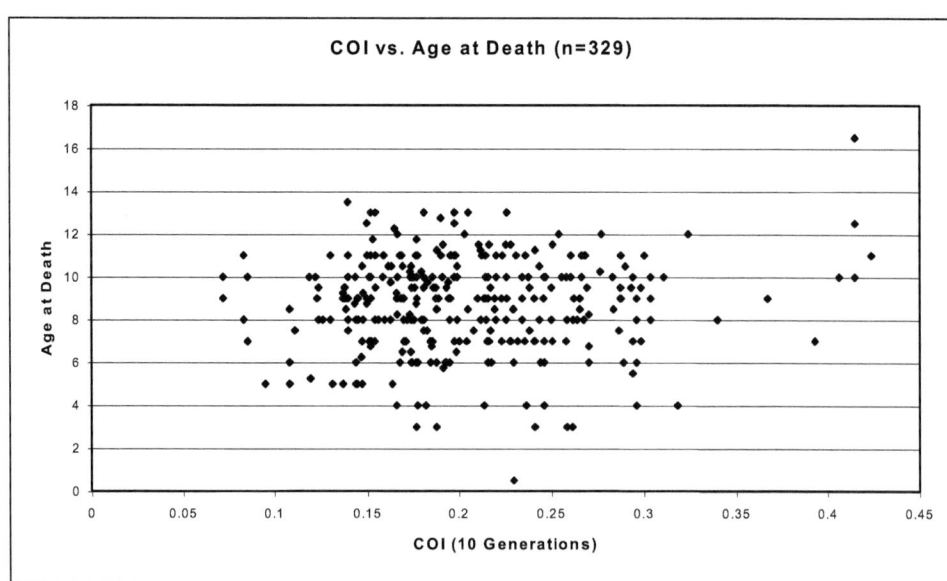

Fig. 5.5: Point diagram of 10-generation inbreeding vs. age at death in Murphy (1991)

5.2.2 Individuals Alive in 1990

5.2.2.1 Population Structure

The Murphy data also include information on n=871 (330 males / 518 females / 23 unknown) dogs that were alive as of Dec 31, 1990 Again, there were significantly fewer males than females in the data (P<0.0001, chi-square=48.15). Birth cohort distribution is rendered in figure 5.6 below:

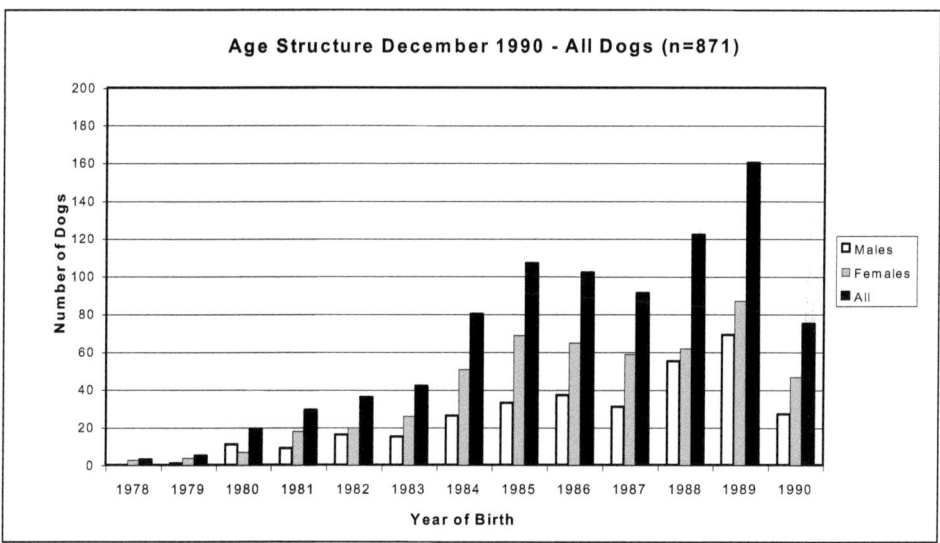

Fig. 5.6: Age structure in UK and IRL Irish Wolfhounds alive in December 1990

5.2.2.2 Age Distribution

As expected, age is not normally distributed within the population (Shapiro-Wilk P<0.0001; Kolmogorov-Smirnov P<0.01). The age distribution of individuals alive in Dec. 1990 is given in table 5.7 below:

Measure	Value (years)
Mean age ± SD	4.13 ± 2.70
Minimum	0.00
5%	0.75
1st quartile	1.75
Median age	3.75
3rd quartile	6.00
95%	9.50
Maximum	12.00

Table 5.7: Statistical parameters for ages of individuals alive in Dec. 1990

5.2.2.3 Gender Effects

No significant effects of gender on age were found in this population (P=0.17, R^2=0.0026, F=1.87, DF=1; type III SS).

5.2.2.4 Inbreeding Effects

Inbreeding Coefficients were calculated from the data of the study at hand, which was possible for 736 individuals (see chapter 6.1.2). There were no significant effects of five, ten or twenty generation Wright's inbreeding coefficients on the age of these dogs; however, Meuwissen's inbreeding coefficients showed a highly significant correlation (P<0.0001, R^2=0.038, F=28.23, DF=1; type III SS. Linear regression coefficient -9.89, SE=1.83).

On the other hand, when the overall population from the same birth cohorts and countries in the data from the present study (see chapter 6.1.2) was examined, it showed that a similar distribution of Meuwissen's coefficients by year of birth existed independently of whether or not the dogs were alive (P<0.0001, R^2=0.014, F=59.38, DF=1. Linear regression coefficient -7.59, SE=0.97)

A diagram of Meuwissen's Inbreeding Coefficients vs. age of the dogs alive in 1990 is rendered in figure 5.7 below.

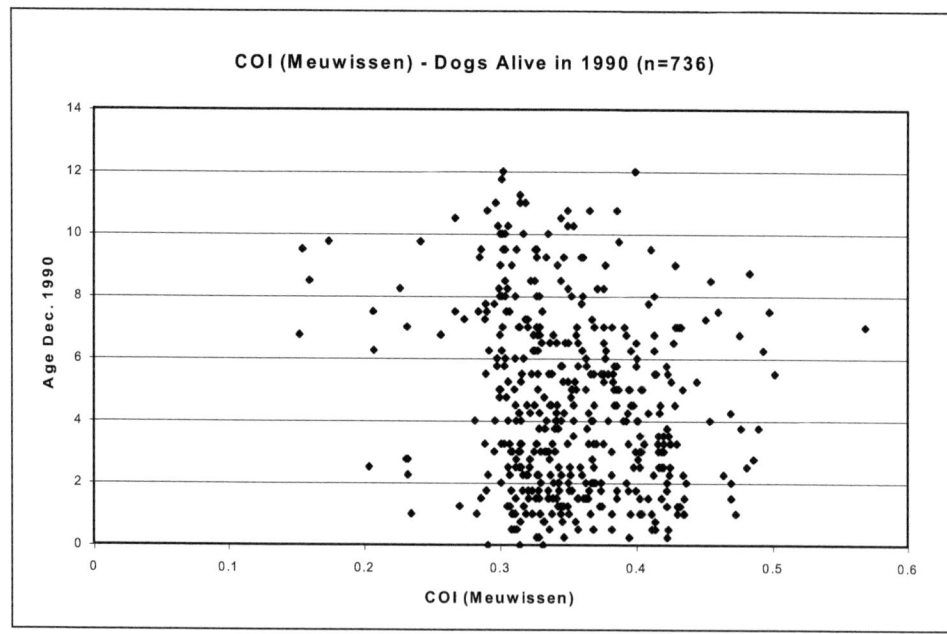

Fig 5.7: *Meuwissen's inbreeding coefficients of dogs alive in 1990*

6 Analysis of the Present Data

6.1 Population Structure and Genetics

6.1.1 Birth Cohorts

As mentioned in chapter 4.1, the population used for the study at hand consisted of n=50'822 Irish Wolfhounds born between 1862 and 2005 (23'219 males / 27'101 females / 502 unknown). There were significantly fewer males than females in the data (P<0.0001, chi-square=299.48). Their distribution by birth cohort is represented in table 6.1 and Fig. 6.1.

Birth Cohort	All	Males	Females	Birth Cohort	All	Males	Females
1862-1900	249	116	131	1960-1969	2301	948	1350
1900-1909	190	91	99	1970-1979	7193	3030	4136
1910-1919	278	137	136	1980-1989	11295	4899	6309
1920-1929	1081	534	547	1990-1999	19410	9356	9960
1930-1939	1231	656	575	2000-2005	3970	1894	1920
1940-1949	764	377	387	Unknown	1817	659	1034
1950-1959	1043	522	517	**Total**	**50822**	**23219**	**27101**

Table 6.1: Distribution of dogs by birth cohort and gender in the database

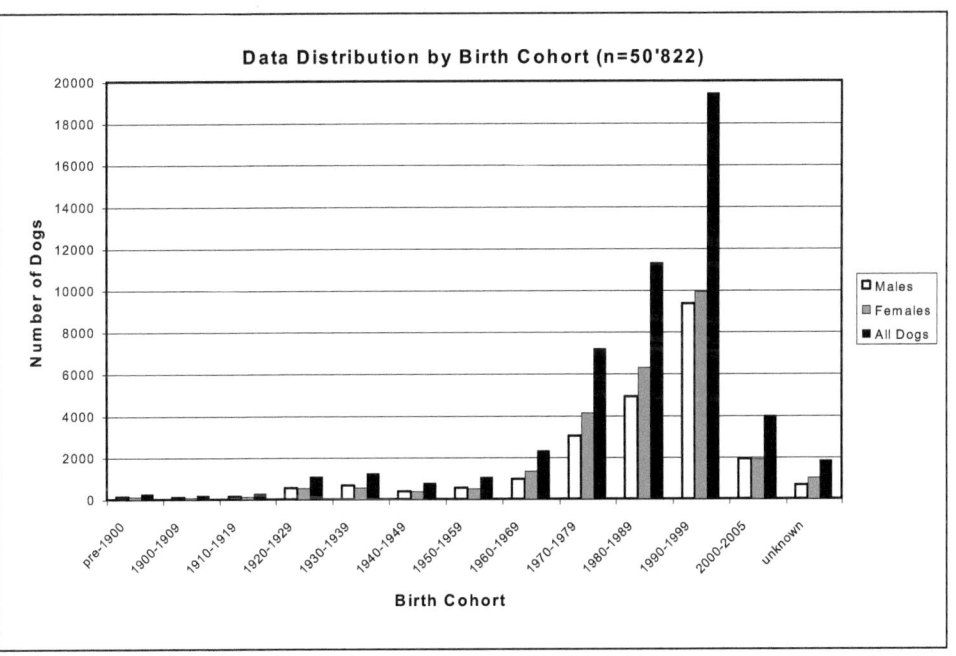

Fig. 6.1: Graphical rendering of Table 6.1

6.1.2 Inbreeding

Four inbreeding coefficients were calculated for all dogs: Wright's Inbreeding Coefficients for 5, 10 and 20 generations, and Meuwissen's inbreeding coefficients back to the beginning of the available data. The distribution of inbreeding coefficients was analysed by class and year of birth. Results are given in table and figure 6.2 below. Figure 6.3 and 6.4 on the next page show the development of Wright's and Meuwissen's inbreeding coefficients in the population over time.

COI Class	5 Generations	10 Generations	20 Generations	Meuwissen
up to 0.05	27002	3114	2452	2469
0.05 to 0.1	11236	6472	679	584
0.1 to 0.15	6199	13837	1663	1537
0.15 to 0.2	3933	13948	3206	1681
0.2 to 0.25	1260	7280	10800	3447
0.25 to 0.3	871	3869	16804	7886
0.3 to 0.35	231	1556	8828	17842
0.35 to 0.4	60	550	4372	9293
0.4 to 0.45	26	145	1419	4297
0.45 to 0.5	4	41	503	1439
0.5 to 0.55	0	10	75	296
above 0.55	0	0	21	51

Table 6.2: *Distribution of different inbreeding coefficient values in the Irish Wolfhound population (n=50'822 dogs).*

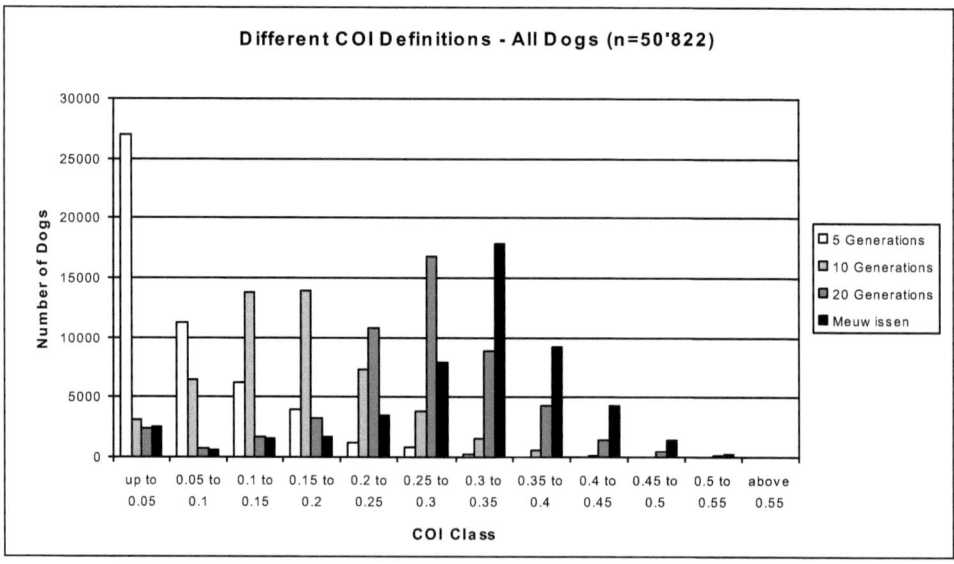

Fig. 6.2: *Graphical rendering of Table 6.2 above*

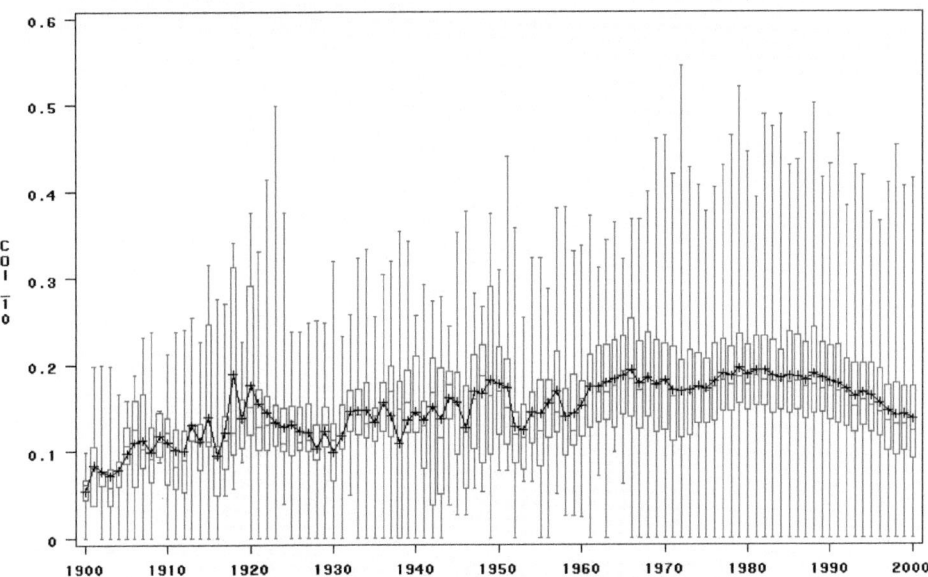
Fig. 6.3: 10-Generation Wright's Inbreeding Coefficients by year of birth

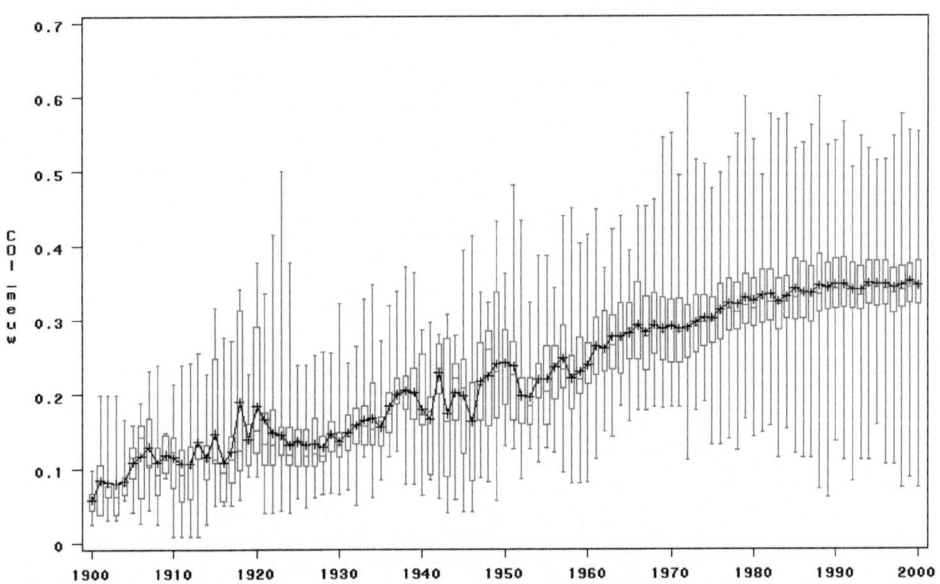
Fig. 6.4: Meuwissen's Inbreeding Coefficients by year of Birth

6.1.3 Geographical Origin

Countries of origin and birth cohorts were distributed as shown in table 6.3 and figure 6.5 below:

	UK/IRL	Continental Europe	North America	Other	Unknown
pre-1900	211	5	0	0	33
1900-1909	146	0	0	0	44
1910-1919	117	6	15	0	140
1920-1929	310	10	87	0	674
1930-1939	134	5	121	3	968
1940-1949	144	0	109	0	511
1950-1959	191	3	218	0	631
1960-1969	762	120	807	2	610
1970-1979	1765	1349	2822	252	1005
1980-1989	3269	3563	2665	704	1094
1990-1999	6236	8177	3275	577	1145
2000-2005	1021	1748	402	130	669
unknown	352	422	126	72	845
Total	**14658**	**15408**	**10647**	**1740**	**8369**

Table 6.3: Distribution of dogs by birth cohorts and countries

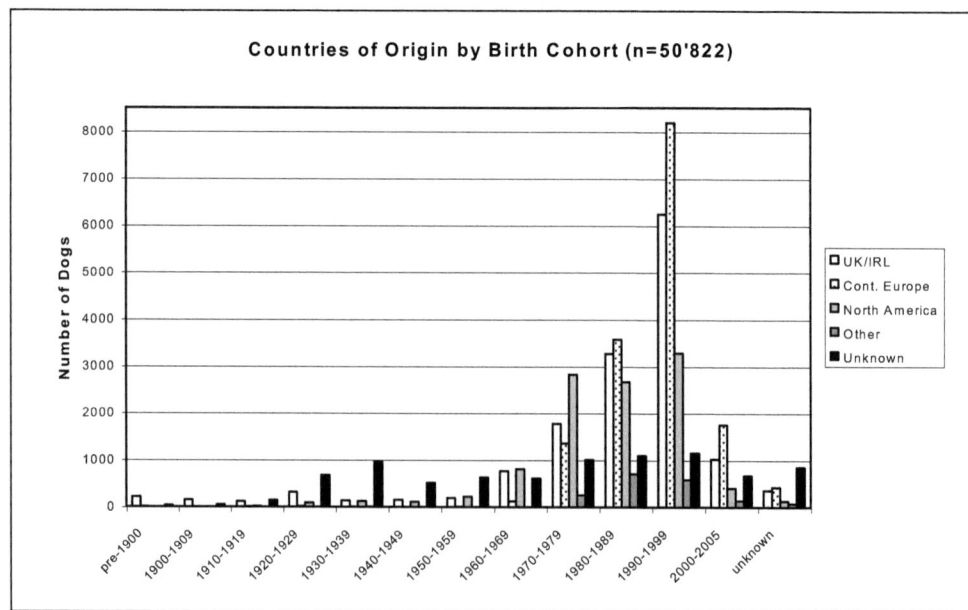

Fig. 6.5: Graphical rendering of table 6.3 above

6.2 Lifespan

Information on lifespan was known for n=1745 individuals. Adjusted for Cohort Bias, n=1423 individuals (583 males / 813 females / 27 unknown) remained. The data contained significantly more females than males (P<0.0001, chi-square=37.89). The lifespan values were not normally distributed (Shapiro-Wilk P<0.0001; Kolmogorov-Smirnow P<0.01). Statistical parameters are rendered in table 6.4 and figure 6.6 below.

Measure	Value (years)
Mean age ± SD	7.84 ± 2.66
Minimum	0.25
5% of dogs dead	3.00
1st quartile	6.00
Median age	8.00
3rd quartile	10.00
95% of dogs dead	12.00
Maximum	16.50

Table 6.4: Statistical measures for lifespan in the overall population

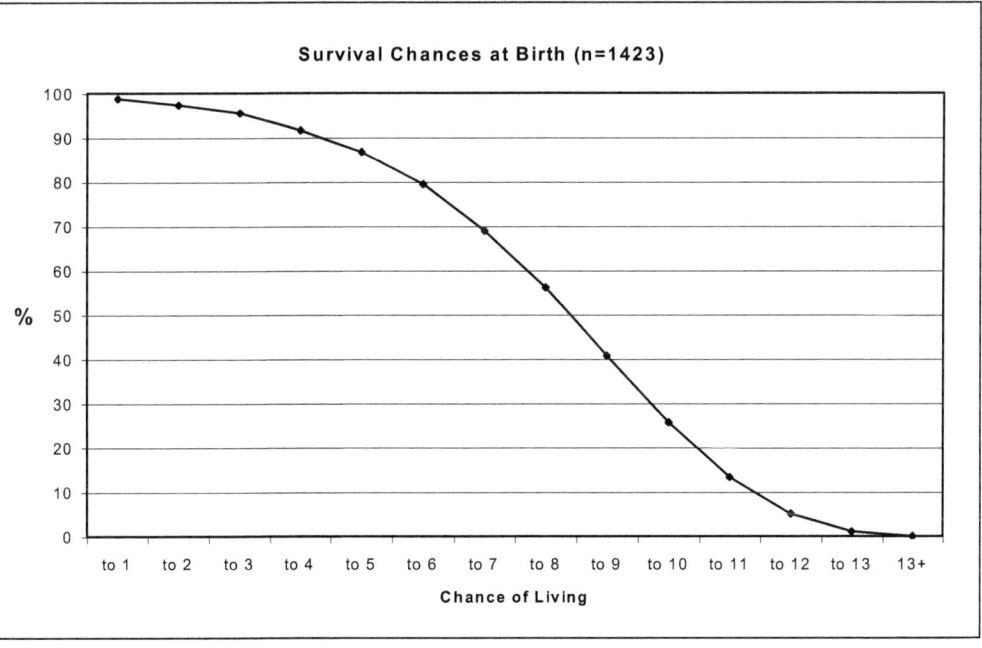

Fig. 6.6: Survival chances at birth, adjusted for Cohort Bias

6.2.1 Data of Living Dogs

Ages at which dogs were still alive were known for n=271 individuals for which no death data were available. Their distribution is rendered in table 6.5:

Measure	Value (years)
Mean age ± SD	8.05 ± 2.17
Minimum	1.84
5%	4.00
1st quartile	6.84
Median age	8.17
3rd quartile	9.67
95%	11.00
Maximum	13.50

Table 6.5: Distribution of dogs known to be alive at certain ages

6.2.2 Causes of Death

6.2.2.1 Adjusted for Cohort Bias

Causes of Death were known for n=468 individuals. Adjusted for Cohort Bias, n=302 individuals remained (148 males / 153 females / 1 unknown). The gender distribution did not significantly differ from an equal distribution model (P=0.77; chi-square=0.083). Causes of death were classified as discussed in chapter 4.3. Their distribution is given in table 6.6:

Cause of Death	n	%	Mean age ± SD
All Dogs	302	100.00	7.84 ± 2.66
GDV	25	8.28	7.09 ± 2.69
DCM	56	18.54	7.11 ± 2.31
OS	58	19.21	6.97 ± 1.87
OCa	54	17.88	7.43 ± 2.43
II	32	10.60	5.04 ± 2.70
Accident	42	13.91	4.85 ± 2.57
OGD	35	11.59	6.21 ± 3.75

Table 6.6: Percentual importance of different causes of death

Based on these data, cause of death was shown to have a highly significant effect on life expectancy (P<0.0001; R^2=0.123, F=6.91, DF=6; type III SS). However, when infectious/ inflammatory diseases and accidental deaths were excluded, no significant effects remained (P=0.28, R^2=0.022, F=1.27, DF=4; type III SS).

6.2.2.2 Influence of Cohort Bias

To assess the influence of Cohort Bias on the percentual frequency of causes of death, the same analysis was carried out in the data that was subject to Cohort Bias. Results are given in table 6.7 below:

Cause of Death	n	%	Mean age ± SD
All Dogs	166	100.00	5.71 ± 2.28
GDV	16	9.64	5.86 ± 2.60
DCM	40	24.10	5.99 ± 1.83
OS	28	16.87	6.37 ± 1.76
OCa	26	15.66	6.20 ± 2.15
II	11	6.63	5.76 ± 2.50
Accident	24	14.46	3.73 ± 2.30
OGD	21	12.65	5.77 ± 2.52

Table 6.7: Dogs subjected to Cohort Bias

Neither the overall distribution of causes of death (P=0.62, chi-square=4.42) nor any of the individual disease distributions did vary significantly between tables 6.6 and 6.7. On the other hand, age of death varied significantly between the two populations as expected (P<0.0014, R^2=0.022, F=10.31, DF=1; type III SS). The distribution of causes of death in the overall population is shown in table 6.8.

Cause of Death	n	%	Mean age ± SD
All Dogs	468	100.00	6.22 ± 2.60*
GDV	41	8.76	6.61 ± 2.69*
DCM	96	20.51	6.65 ± 2.19*
OS	86	18.38	6.77 ± 1.85*
OCa	80	17.09	7.04 ± 2.40*
II	43	9.19	5.22 ± 2.64*
Accident	66	14.10	4.45 ± 2.52*
OGD	56	11.97	6.05 ± 3.32*

Table 6.8: Distribution of causes of death in the overall population. *Mean age ± SD is tainted with Cohort Bias in this table.

6.2.3 Inbreeding Effects

6.2.3.1 Lifespan

No significant effects of 5-, 10- and 20-generation Wright's inbreeding coefficients as well as Meuwissen's inbreeding coefficient on age at death were found in the present data. Although the latter was borderline, R^2 remains very low. The effects described in chapter 5.2.2.4 should also be taken into account as a possible source of interaction in this case. Table 6.9 and figure 6.7 on the following page show the lack of correlation found in this analysis.

Coefficient	R^2	p	F	Coefficient	R^2	p	F
5 Gens	0.000037	0.82	0.05	20 Gens	0.0013	0.18	1.81
10 Gens	0.000045	0.80	0.06	Meuwissen	0.0026	0.06	3.53

Table 6.9: Influence of inbreeding on lifespan (n=1423; DF=1; type III SS)

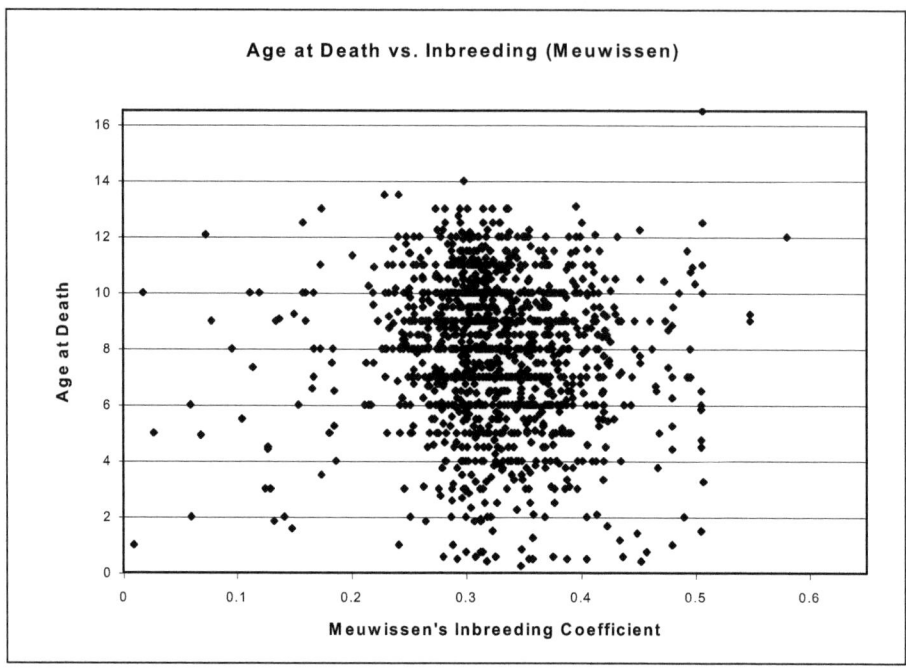

Fig. 6.7: Diagram of measured lifespan and Meuwissen's Inbreeding Coefficients, adjusted for Cohort Bias. No significant correlation was found.

6.2.3.2 Causes of Death

Since an association of increasing inbreeding coefficients with DCM in Irish Wolfhounds has been reported in the literature (Broschk 2004), this possibility was also analysed in our population. Inbreeding levels in the population affected with DCM and the randomly chosen reference population (see chapter 4.5) were not significantly different for 5- and 10-generation Wright's inbreeding coefficients as well as Meuwissen's inbreeding coefficients. On the other hand, 20-generation Wright's inbreeding coefficients were significantly lower in dogs affected with DCM than in dogs without DCM, but R^2 remains very low (0.26 ± 0.09 vs. 0.28 ± 0.07; P=0.033, R^2=0.0014, F=4.54; Type III SS).

6.2.4 Gender Effects

6.2.4.1 Lifespan

Lifespan data adjusted for Cohort Bias are given in table 6.10. Again, females lived significantly longer than males ($P<0.0001$, $R^2=0.025$, $F=35.42$, $DF=1$; type III SS).

Group	n	Mean Age ± SD
All Dogs	1423	7.84 ± 2.66
Males	583	7.34 ± 2.73
Females	813	8.18 ± 2.52

Table 6.10: Lifespan data adjusted for Cohort Bias

6.2.4.2 Causes of Death

When only animals with known causes of death were considered and Cohort Bias removed, 302 individuals (148 males / 153 females / 1 unknown) remained for analysis. Lifespan results for this population are given in table 6.11:

Group	n	Mean Age ± SD
All Dogs	302	6.50 ± 2.72
Males	148	6.10 ± 2.74
Females	153	6.91 ± 2.65

Table 6.11: Lifespan of Dogs with known causes of death, adjusted for Cohort Bias

As in the Bernardi/Prokopenko data (see chapter 5.1.5.2), males were found to be at an increased risk for death by DCM (24.3% of male deaths as opposed to 13.1% of female deaths; $P=0.012$, chi-square=6.29; $P=0.017$; Fisher's two-sided test), and females were found to be at an increased risk for death by cancer other than osteogenic sarcoma (8.8% of male deaths as opposed to 26.1% of female deaths; $P<0.0001$, chi-square=15.63; $P=0.0007$; Fisher's two-sided test). No significant gender effects were found for the other disease classes.

Based on the results presented in chapter 6.2.1.2, the influence of gender on cause of death was also studied in the data not adjusted for Cohort Bias. The results remained identical for all disease classes (DCM: 27.16% vs. 14.04%; $P=0.0005$, chi-square=12.29; $P=0.00054$, Fisher's two-sided test. Cancer other than OS: 12.50% vs. 21.28%; $P=0.011$, chi-square=6.40; $P=0.013$, Fisher's two-sided test).

Given that no information on castration status was available, it was impossible to test the influence of castration on cause of death and life expectancy in this population.

6.2.5 Effects of Popular Sires

Popular sires were defined as individuals of which lifespan of 10 or more first generation progeny was known in the data adjusted for Cohort Bias. This resulted in n=197 individuals with 13 different sires. Lifespan of these dogs by sire is rendered in figure 6.8 on the next page. Only one female in the database had more than 10 such progeny; therefore, no analysis of popular dam effects could be carried out.

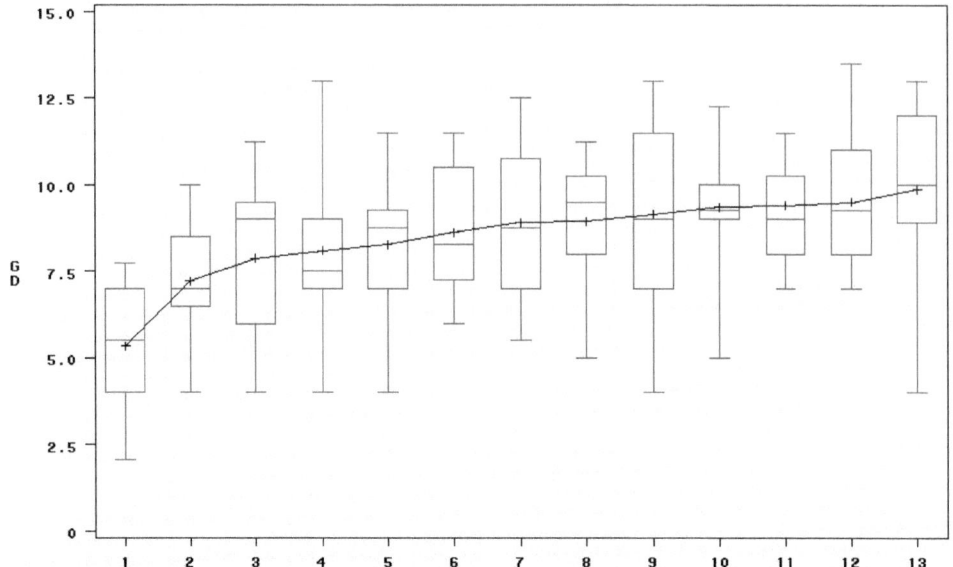

Fig. 6.8: Lifespan (GD) of direct progeny of sires with 10 or more first-generation descendants with known lifespan (n=197)

The number of descendants of known lifespan was also compared to the total number of known descendants in the population adjusted for Cohort Bias. The popular sires were thus divided as shown in table 6.12. The "Known Progeny" category refers to the known number of direct progeny of the sire in the database as 100%, which may be too low.

Sire	Year of Birth	Country	Known Progeny	Mean age ± SD	Age of Sire
1	1980	UK	15 of 40 (37.5%)	5.34 ± 1.74	7.75
2	1976	UK	13 of 35 (37.1%)	7.21 ± 1.67	5
3	1976	Ireland	13 of 49 (26.5%)	7.87 ± 2.20	10.25
4	1959	UK	10 of 34 (29.4%)	8.10 ± 2.47	6
5	1974	UK	31 of 83 (37.4%)	8.26 ± 1.86	8.75
6	1975	UK	16 of 46 (34.8%)	8.63 ± 1.88	9.5
7	1966	UK	12 of 42 (28.6%)	8.92 ± 2.30	9.75
8	1971	Ireland	13 of 86 (15.1%)	8.94 ± 2.12	>6
9	1961	UK	10 of 34 (29.4%)	9.15 ± 2.85	unknown
10*	1976	Ireland	14 of 34 (41.2%)	9.36 ± 1.67	11.25
11	1969	UK	13 of 53 (24.5%)	9.40 ± 1.44	9
12**	1963	Ireland	10 of 71 (14.1%)	9.50 ± 2.19	unknown
13	1970	UK	27 of 72 (37.5%)	9.86 ± 2.25	8.75

Table 6.12: Popular sires in the data. *son of 8; **son of 4

These lifespan distributions varied significantly between the progeny of different sires (P<0.0001, R^2=0.26, F=5.38, DF=12; type III SS). Progeny of sires 1 and 2 contrasted significantly with the progeny of other sires (P<0.0001, R^2=0.25, F=42.63) However, when sires 1 and 2 were excluded, no significant sire effect remained (P=0.12, R^2=0.091, F=1.58, DF=10; type III SS).

6.2.6 Effects of Birth Cohort

Effects of birth cohort were also investigated as a possible influence on lifespan over time. Due to the small numbers of dogs available before 1960, data from these individuals were merged into one category as given in table 6.13.

Birth Cohort	Number of Dogs	Mean Age ± SD
Pre-1900	5	5.80 ± 3.35
1900-1909	3	5.67 ± 3.06
1910-1919	4	5.63 ± 3.68
1920-1929	10	5.68 ± 2.50
1930-1939	5	4.90 ± 3.36
1940-1949	8	6.78 ± 2.74
1950-1959	22	7.98 ± 2.58
Pre-1960	**57**	**6.66 ± 2.90**
1960-1969	**113**	**8.92 ± 2.23**
1970-1979	**486**	**8.24 ± 2.48**
1980-1989	**523**	**7.59 ± 2.68**
1990-1993	**210**	**7.46 ± 2.53**
Unknown	34	7.10 ± 3.37

Table 6.13: Lifespan by birth cohort

Statistical analysis of the categories marked in bold showed a highly significant influence of birth cohort on lifespan (P<0.0001; R^2=0.039, F=13.99, DF=4; type III SS), which shows a steady decrease in life expectancy in the population born after the 1960s.

6.2.7 Generalised Linear Models

Generalised Linear Models were designed for the overall death data with the goal of explaining as much of the existing variance as possible. Since death data were not normally distributed, type III SS p-values were chosen in all cases. Where specified, birth cohorts pre-1970 were merged as shown in table 6.13. The results are given in table 6.14 on the following page.

	UC Excluded – Birth Cohorts Merged			UC Included – Birth Cohorts Merged			UC Included – Birth Cohorts not Merged		
n in Model	267			1329			1329		
n Excluded	75			94			94		
R-square	0.3848			0.2298			0.2521		
	DF	p	F	DF	p	F	DF	p	F
Model	36	<0.0001	4.00	52	<0.0001	7.32	69	<0.0001	6.15
CoD	6	0.0002	4.66	7	<0.0001	14.36	7	<0.0001	14.09
Gender	1	0.026	5.02	1	<0.0001	25.59	1	<0.0001	28.07
BC	3	0.0022	5.02	4	0.0003	5.33	11	0.0007	2.96
CC	NI	NI	NI	3	0.0056	4.22	3	0.0073	4.02
CoD*CC	21	<0.0001	3.88	21	<0.0001	4.21	21	<0.0001	4.44
BC*CC	NI	NI	NI	11	0.0002	3.27	14	0.0003	2.87
Meuw*BC	NI	NI	NI	4	<0.0001	8.04	12	0.0016	2.65
Meuw*Gender	1	0.0071	7.37	NI	NI	NI	NI	NI	NI
Meuw*CC	3	0.0021	5.03	NI	NI	NI	NI	NI	NI

Table 6.14: Generalised Linear Models with type III SS for the overall population. UC=unknown causes of death; n=number of dogs; DF=Degrees of Freedom; CoD=Cause of Death (see chapter 4.3); CC=Country Class (see chapter 6.1.3); BC=Birth Cohort (see chapters 6.1.3 and 6.2.6 for discussion of merging – Dogs born after 1993 excluded); Meuw=Meuwissen's Inbreeding Coefficient; NI=not included (non-significant p values); * = Interaction of Variables.

6.3 Population Genetics of Dogs Born 1965 and After

6.3.1 Inbreeding

The population of dogs born 1965 and after was studied for its genetic composition, as well as for founders of diseases presumed hereditary. The distribution of inbreeding coefficients is rendered in table 6.15 and figure 6.9 below. Their development over time is rendered in fig. 6.10 and 6.11 on the following page.

Inbreeding	COI (5)	COI (10)	COI (20)	Meuwissen's IC
up to 0.05	23044	1296	732	762
0.05-0.1	9414	5553	172	63
0.1 to 0.15	5257	11699	330	221
0.15 to 0.2	3552	12591	1980	486
0.2 to 0.25	1078	6512	9559	2320
0.25 to 0.3	777	3614	16044	7162
0.3 to 0.35	209	1442	8396	17290
0.35 to 0.4	51	522	4239	9111
0.4 to 0.45	20	130	1370	4227
0.45 to 0.5	4	37	495	1425
0.5 to 0.55	0	10	69	289
above 0.55	0	0	20	50

Table 6.15: Distribution of inbreeding coefficients in Irish Wolfhounds born post-1964. COI (n) = Wright's Inbreeding Coefficient over n generations

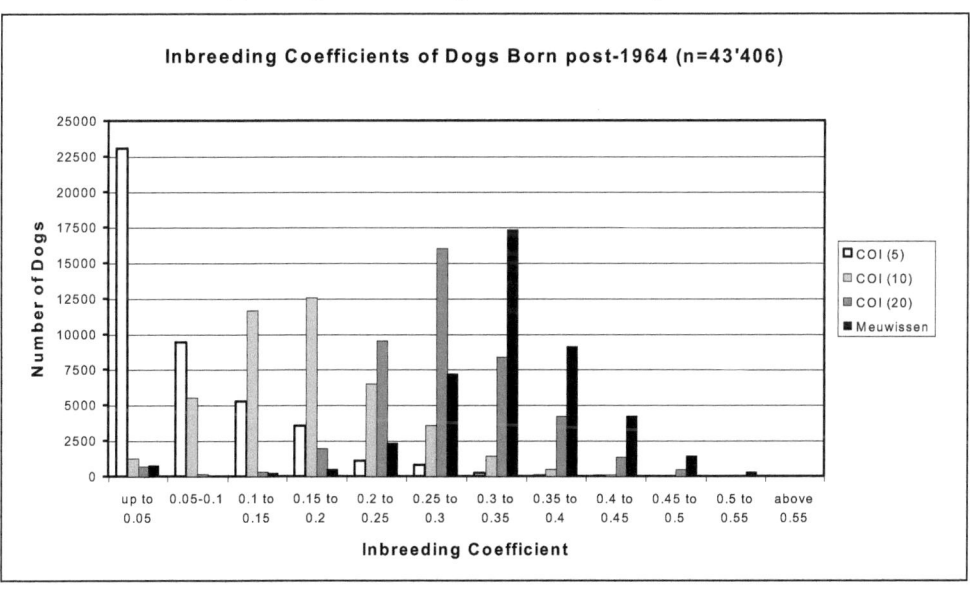

Fig. 6.9: Distribution of inbreeding coefficients in Irish Wolfhounds born post-1964.

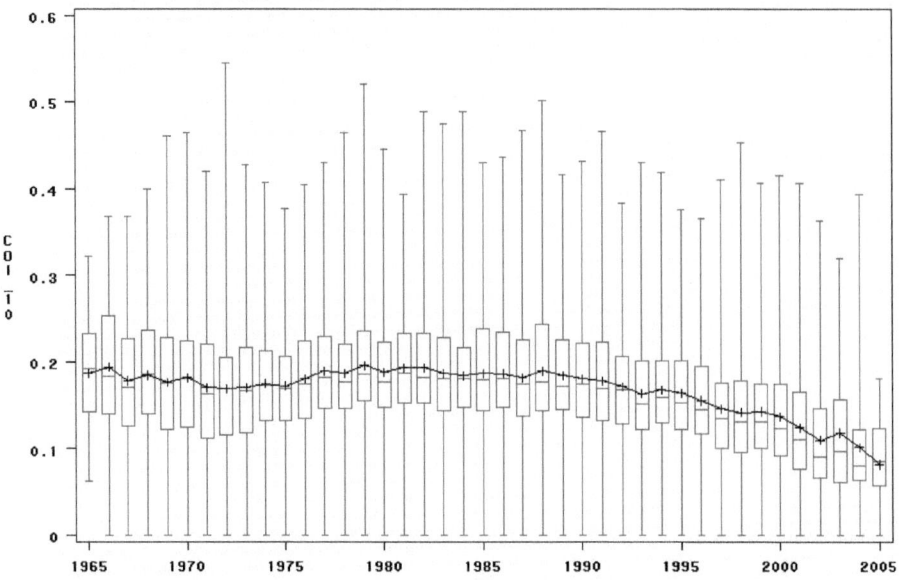

Fig. 6.10: *10-Generation Wright's Inbreeding Coefficients by year of birth*

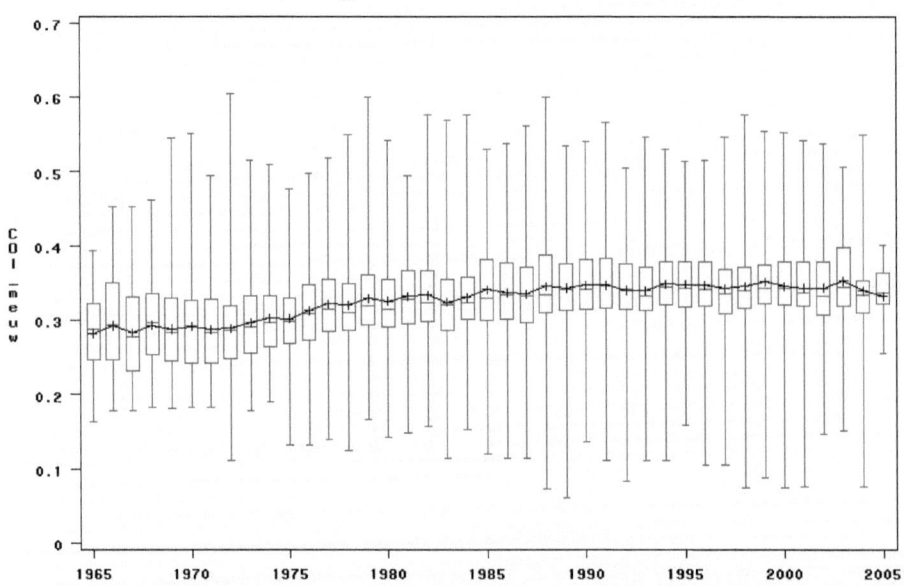

Fig. 6.11: *Meuwissen's Inbreeding Coefficients by year of birth*

6.3.2 Ancestor Analysis

6.3.2.1 Whole Database

Ancestor analysis was performed with the prob_orig.exe program of the PEDIG package, determining the 20 most important ancestors of the population born from 1965 to 2005, going back all the way to the beginning of the available data. This resulted in table 6.16 below:

Rank	Dog ID	sex	YoB	Contribution	Cumulative	Progeny	Country
1	5838	m	1951	0.2602	0.2602	15	US to UK
2	4732	m	1939	0.1972	0.4574	10	UK
3	4703	f	1939	0.1045	0.5619	4	UK
4	5538	m	1949	0.0792	0.6411	11	US
5	4605	f	1938	0.0786	0.7197	4	UK
6	5184	m	1944	0.0706	0.7903	3	UK
7	5252	f	1945	0.0402	0.8305	2	IRL
8	4681	f	1938	0.0291	0.8596	2	UK
9	4475	f	1937	0.0239	0.8835	1	UK
10	4820	f	1939	0.0202	0.9037	3	UK
11	3132	m	1927	0.0132	0.9169	13	UK to US
12	5385	m	1947	0.0106	0.9275	5	US
13	5045	m	1943	0.0080	0.9355	7	US
14	4794	m	1939	0.0066	0.9421	5	US
15	5273	f	1946	0.0055	0.9476	1	UK
16	5541	f	1949	0.0049	0.9525	2	US
17	1900	m	1889	0.0030	0.9555	8	UK
18	1949	m	1893	0.0028	0.9583	6	UK
19	2015	m	1896	0.0025	0.9608	9	UK
20	1940	f	1892	0.0025	0.9633	5	UK

Table 6.16: Genetic contribution of the top 20 ancestors on the population. YoB=Year of Birth. Progeny=number of direct 1st generation progeny in the database. US=United States, UK=United Kingdom, IRL=Republic of Ireland. Dog 1 was born in the US and exported to the UK, while the reverse is true in the case of dog 11.

Reading example: The dog ranked as the 4th most important ancestor, ID-Nr. 5538, male, born 1949, contributed 0.0792 (i.e. 7.92%) to the gene pool of the Irish Wolfhound population born 1965-2005. Cumulatively, the first four dogs explain 0.6411 (i.e. 64.11%) of genetic variability in this population. The dog had 11 direct 1st generation progeny in the database and was born in the United States of America.

It is remarkable that despite the fact that this table was calculated all the way back to the first dogs in the database (from 1862 onwards), the top ten ancestors that account for over 90% of genetic variability altogether were all born between 1937 and 1951. Also, with the exception of individuals 7 (4 generations complete, then 3 missing dogs accounting for 25% of the pedigree) and 8 (3 generations on sire's side, but dam's side complete), all of the top 10 ancestors can be tracked back for at least 10 generations.

The individual and cumulative contributions of the twenty most important ancestors to the gene pool of the reference population are rendered graphically in figure 6.12 below:

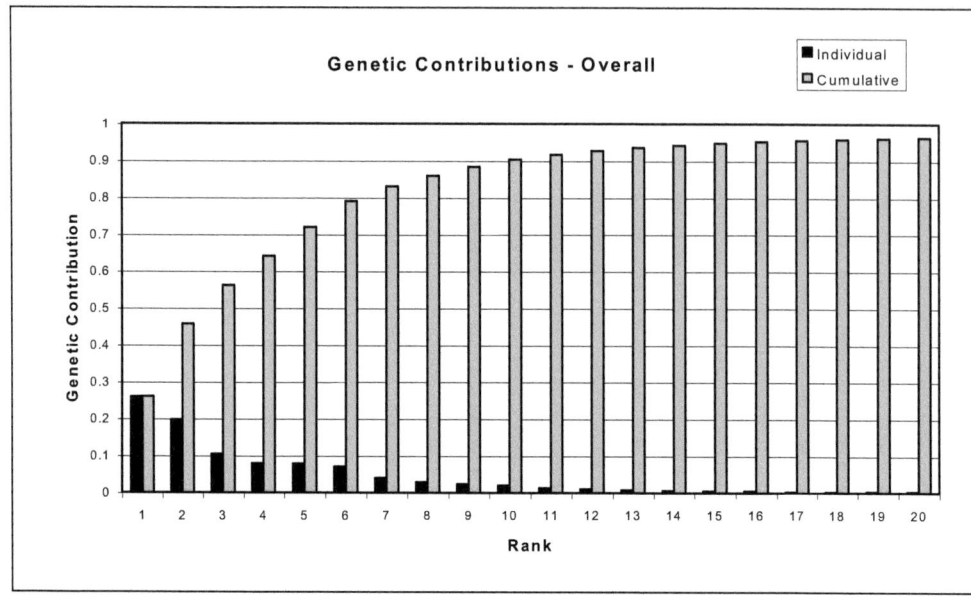

Fig. 6.12: Graphical rendering of table 6.16

These results demonstrate that over 25% of genetic variability in the Irish Wolfhound population born between 1965 and 2005 can be explained by one ancestor, over 50% by three ancestors, over 75% by six ancestors, and over 90% by ten ancestors only.

6.3.2.2 10 Generations

The same ancestor analysis was also performed for the population of dogs born 1965-2005, this time calculating back for 10 generations instead of the whole database. The results are presented in table 6.17 below:

Rank	Dog ID	sex	YoB	Contribution	Cumulative	Progeny	Country
1	5838	m	1951	0.2602	0.2602	15	US to UK
2	4732	m	1939	0.1972	0.4574	10	UK
3	4703	f	1939	0.1045	0.5619	4	UK
4	5538	m	1949	0.0792	0.6411	11	US
5	4605	m	1938	0.0786	0.7197	4	UK
6	5184	m	1944	0.0706	0.7903	3	UK
7	5252	f	1945	0.0402	0.8305	2	IRL
8	4681	f	1938	0.0291	0.8596	2	UK
9	4475	f	1937	0.0239	0.8835	1	UK
10	4820	f	1939	0.0202	0.9037	3	UK
11	3132	m	1927	0.0132	0.9169	13	UK to US
12	5385	m	1947	0.0106	0.9275	5	US
13	5045	m	1943	0.0080	0.9355	7	US
14	4794	m	1939	0.0066	0.9421	5	US
15	5273	f	1946	0.0055	0.9476	1	UK
16	5541	f	1949	0.0049	0.9525	2	US
17	5283	f	1946	0.0030	0.9555	1	US
18	5548	m	1949	0.0030	0.9585	1	IRL
19	4552	f	1938	0.0028	0.9613	3	US
20	5328	f	1946	0.0025	0.9638	1	US

Table 6.17: Genetic contribution of the top 20 ancestors to the population born 1965 to 2005, calculated over 10 generations. Reading is analogous to table 6.16.

It is noteworthy that the only differences between tables 6.16 and 6.17 can be found amongst ranks 17 to 20 in this calculation.

6.4 Ancestor Analyses of Diseases Presumed Hereditary

It was decided to also run the ancestor analyses on individuals affected with four diseases presumed hereditary: Dilatative Cardiomyopathy, Osteogenic Sarcoma, Gastric Dilation Volvulus, and Portosystemic Shunt. These diseases were chosen based on the comparably large number of confirmed cases in the overall database as well as the findings of the literature review (see chapter 3).

The analysis consisted of ancestor analysis similar to what is described in chapter 6.3.2. The 20 most important ancestors and their percentual contributions were calculated for both the population of affected dogs and a randomly chosen reference population of identical countries of origin and years of birth. The results of the two ancestor analyses were then compared. See chapter 4.3.2 for a more detailed description of how the reference populations were created.

While this method does not allow an exact determination of the mode of inheritance, it has the advantage that heredity in itself can be detected without health data on complete litters being necessary for the calculation.

No notable differences were found for any of the diseases when calculating back to the beginning of the database – these results are not displayed in this chapter, which is limited to the results found when calculating back 10 generations. A table of all rankings including calculations back to the beginning of the database can be found in the appendix.

An overview of the analysed data is given in table 6.18 below:

Disease	Number of Individuals
Dilated Cardiomyopathy	160
Osteogenic Sarcoma	82
Gastric Dilation Volvulus	47
Portosystemic Shunt	20

Table 6.18*: Disease cases available for ancestor analysis. The differences in available cases to the findings presented in the previous chapters is due to the inclusion of both data subject to Cohort Bias and data of affected dogs of which no death data is known*

As shown in this table, we had confirmed information of n=20 Irish Wolfhound litters (born 1976-2004) in which PSS had occurred. While there were not enough PSS cases in the database to warrant a separate category for the previous analyses (where PSS was classified as category 7, "Other General Debilitation"), it was decided to also subject these data to ancestor analysis.

It is interesting to note that while there are obvious differences between the reference and affected populations of the first three death classes, these differences are strikingly similar in all three diseases. On the other hand, the marked discrepancies between the two populations for portosystemic shunt did not exhibit similarities to those between the other groups.

6.4.1 Dilatative Cardiomyopathy

6.4.1.1 Reference Population

ID	Rank	sex	YoB	Contribution	Cumulative	Progeny	Country
5838	1	m	1951	0.2533	0.2533	15	US to UK
4732	2	m	1939	0.1970	0.4503	10	UK
4703	3	f	1939	0.1029	0.5532	4	UK
4605	4	f	1938	0.0772	0.6304	4	UK
5538	5	m	1949	0.0764	0.7068	10	US
5184	6	m	1944	0.0687	0.7755	3	UK
5252	7	f	1945	0.0407	0.8162	2	IRL
4681	8	f	1938	0.0302	0.8464	2	UK
4475	9	f	1937	0.0240	0.8704	1	UK
4820	10	f	1939	0.0197	0.8901	3	UK
6476	11	m	1958	0.0172	0.9073	18	US
6620	12	f	1959	0.0122	0.9195	13	US
5385	13	m	1947	0.0090	0.9285	5	US
5045	14	m	1943	0.0083	0.9368	6	US
4794	15	f	1939	0.0066	0.9434	5	US
5273	16	f	1946	0.0054	0.9488	1	UK
5541	17	f	1949	0.0040	0.9528	2	US
6378	18	f	1957	0.0034	0.9562	1	IRL
5548	19	m	1949	0.0029	0.9591	1	IRL
5117	20	f	1944	0.0029	0.9620	3	US

Table 6.19: Reference population results for DCM. Reading is analogous to table 6.16.

6.4.1.2 Affected Dogs

ID	Rank	sex	YoB	Contribution	Cumulative	Progeny	Country
5838	1	m	1951	0.1668	0.1668	14	US to UK
6261	2	m	1955	0.0753	0.2421	9	UK
5561	3	f	1949	0.0641	0.3062	4	UK
5349	4	f	1946	0.0586	0.3648	3	UK
7978	5	m	1967	0.0332	0.3980	13	UK
8251	6	f	1968	0.0312	0.4292	6	IRL
8847	7	m	1969	0.0286	0.4578	22	UK
5510	8	f	1948	0.0275	0.4853	2	UK
5538	9	m	1949	0.0219	0.5072	10	US
6707	10	m	1960	0.0187	0.5259	13	UK
6660	11	f	1960	0.0175	0.5434	6	IRL
6661	12	f	1960	0.0149	0.5583	7	IRL to UK
6620	13	f	1959	0.0146	0.5729	11	US
7174	14	f	1963	0.0138	0.5867	2	UK
6744	15	f	1961	0.0117	0.5984	9	IRL
6180	16	f	1955	0.0115	0.6099	5	IRL
6100	17	m	1954	0.0114	0.6213	4	IRL
8444	18	f	1968	0.0108	0.6321	10	UK
7791	19	m	1966	0.0106	0.6427	7	UK
6755	20	m	1961	0.0096	0.6523	10	IRL

Table 6.20: Affected population results for DCM. Reading is analogous to table 6.16.

6.4.2 Osteogenic Sarcoma

6.4.2.1 Reference Population

ID	Rank	sex	YoB	Contribution	Cumulative	Progeny	Country
5838	1	m	1951	0.2387	0.2387	15	US to UK
4732	2	m	1939	0.1921	0.4308	10	UK
4703	3	f	1939	0.0990	0.5298	4	UK
4605	4	f	1938	0.0745	0.6043	4	UK
5538	5	m	1949	0.0639	0.6682	9	US
5184	6	m	1944	0.0639	0.7321	3	UK
5252	7	f	1945	0.0416	0.7737	2	IRL
4681	8	f	1938	0.0313	0.8050	2	UK
4475	9	f	1937	0.0229	0.8279	1	UK
6476	10	m	1958	0.0216	0.8495	19	US
6874	11	f	1961	0.0184	0.8679	6	UK
4820	12	f	1939	0.0164	0.8843	3	UK
6620	13	f	1959	0.0149	0.8992	12	US
5385	14	m	1947	0.0106	0.9098	5	US
5045	15	m	1943	0.0100	0.9198	6	US
4794	16	m	1939	0.0078	0.9276	5	US
5273	17	f	1946	0.0056	0.9332	1	UK
5541	18	f	1949	0.0050	0.9382	2	US
6998	19	f	1962	0.0045	0.9427	1	UK
6378	20	f	1957	0.0043	0.9470	1	IRL

Table 6.21: Reference population results for OS. Reading is analogous to table 6.16.

6.4.2.2 Affected Dogs

ID	Rank	sex	YoB	Contribution	Cumulative	Progeny	Country
5838	1	m	1951	0.1929	0.1929	14	US to UK
6261	2	m	1955	0.0777	0.2706	9	UK
5561	3	f	1949	0.0720	0.3426	4	UK
5349	4	f	1946	0.0616	0.4042	3	UK
6135	5	f	1954	0.0329	0.4371	11	UK
5510	6	f	1948	0.0303	0.4674	2	UK
6476	7	m	1958	0.0289	0.4963	16	US
6707	8	m	1960	0.0269	0.5232	13	US
5538	9	m	1949	0.0263	0.5495	10	US
8251	10	f	1968	0.0245	0.5740	5	IRL
6620	11	f	1959	0.0218	0.5958	11	US
7326	12	m	1964	0.0206	0.6164	18	IRL
7002	13	m	1962	0.0178	0.6342	15	UK
8444	14	f	1968	0.0157	0.6499	10	UK
7052	15	m	1963	0.0146	0.6645	15	IRL
6744	16	f	1961	0.0114	0.6759	8	IRL
5625	17	m	1950	0.0113	0.6872	4	IRL
6661	18	f	1960	0.0108	0.6980	7	IRL to UK
7068	19	f	1963	0.0093	0.7073	3	UK
5488	20	f	1948	0.0082	0.7155	3	UK

Table 6.22: Affected population results for OS. Reading is analogous to table 6.16.

6.4.3 Gastric Dilation Volvulus

6.4.3.1 Reference Population

ID	Rank	sex	YoB	Contribution	Cumulative	Progeny	Country
4732	1	m	1939	0.1516	0.1516	10	UK
5838	2	m	1951	0.1453	0.2969	15	US to UK
6636	3	m	1959	0.1205	0.4174	21	UK
4605	4	f	1938	0.0584	0.4758	4	UK
4703	5	f	1939	0.0537	0.5295	4	UK
5538	6	m	1949	0.0452	0.5747	8	US
5184	7	m	1944	0.0341	0.6088	3	UK
4681	8	f	1938	0.0290	0.6378	2	UK
5252	9	f	1945	0.0288	0.6666	2	IRL
6476	10	m	1958	0.0229	0.6895	18	US
6707	11	m	1960	0.0222	0.7117	21	US
4475	12	f	1937	0.0183	0.7300	1	UK
7326	13	m	1964	0.0164	0.7464	23	IRL
6620	14	f	1959	0.0151	0.7615	12	US
6640	15	f	1959	0.0125	0.7740	4	UK
6544	16	m	1958	0.0099	0.7839	7	UK
7052	17	m	1963	0.0096	0.7935	23	IRL
7239	18	f	1964	0.0092	0.8027	5	UK
5045	19	m	1943	0.0091	0.8118	6	US
7051	20	m	1963	0.0089	0.8207	13	IRL

Table 6.23: *Reference population results for GVD. Reading is analogous to table 6.16.*

6.4.3.2 Affected Dogs

ID	Rank	sex	YoB	Contribution	Cumulative	Progeny	Country
5838	1	m	1951	0.1813	0.1813	13	US to UK
6261	2	m	1955	0.0745	0.2558	9	UK
5561	3	f	1949	0.0694	0.3252	4	UK
5349	4	f	1946	0.0638	0.3890	3	UK
5510	5	f	1948	0.0327	0.4217	2	UK
8251	6	f	1968	0.0252	0.4469	4	IRL
5538	7	m	1949	0.0249	0.4718	10	US
7326	8	m	1964	0.0245	0.4963	17	IRL
7052	9	m	1963	0.0215	0.5178	15	IRL
6476	10	m	1958	0.0203	0.5381	14	US
7002	11	m	1962	0.0177	0.5558	12	UK
6620	12	f	1959	0.0157	0.5715	10	US
6750	13	f	1961	0.0154	0.5869	7	IRL to UK
6661	14	f	1960	0.0150	0.6019	5	IRL to UK
7174	15	f	1963	0.0112	0.6131	3	UK
7051	16	m	1963	0.0110	0.6241	6	IRL
6177	17	f	1955	0.0108	0.6349	1	US
6747	18	m	1961	0.0100	0.6449	5	IRL
6555	19	m	1959	0.0092	0.6541	8	US
8444	20	f	1968	0.0089	0.6630	6	UK

Table 6.23: *Affected population results for GDV. Reading is analogous to table 6.16.*

6.4.4 Portosystemic Shunt

6.4.4.1 Reference Population

ID	Rank	sex	YoB	Contribution	Cumulative	Progeny	Country
5838	1	m	1951	0.2118	0.2118	14	US to UK
5561	2	f	1949	0.0904	0.3022	4	UK
6261	3	m	1955	0.0891	0.3913	10	UK
5349	4	f	1946	0.0673	0.4586	3	UK
5510	5	f	1948	0.0291	0.4877	2	UK
8251	6	f	1968	0.0271	0.5148	7	IRL
7719	7	m	1966	0.0251	0.5399	18	UK
6135	8	f	1954	0.0247	0.5646	11	UK
5538	9	m	1949	0.0205	0.5851	9	US
6476	10	m	1958	0.0203	0.6054	17	US
7617	11	m	1966	0.0161	0.6215	15	IRL
6620	12	f	1959	0.0160	0.6375	11	US
5046	13	m	1943	0.0144	0.6519	3	UK to IRL
7310	14	f	1964	0.0139	0.6658	2	UK
11392	15	m	1973	0.0114	0.6772	26	US
6684	16	m	1960	0.0111	0.6883	15	IRL
5803	17	f	1951	0.0094	0.6977	5	UK
7677	18	m	1966	0.0090	0.7067	11	UK
9386	19	m	1970	0.0079	0.7146	5	US
8444	20	f	1968	0.0076	0.7222	10	UK

Table 6.25: Reference population results for PSS. Reading is analogous to table 6.16.

6.4.4.2 Affected Dogs

ID	Rank	sex	YoB	Contribution	Cumulative	Progeny	Country
6844	1	m	1961	0.0610	0.0610	16	UK
9249	2	m	1970	0.0516	0.1126	20	UK
12386	3	m	1975	0.0426	0.1552	15	UK
10369	4	m	1972	0.0300	0.1852	7	UK
10362	5	f	1972	0.0252	0.2104	6	UK
11392	6	m	1973	0.0239	0.2343	13	US
7978	7	m	1967	0.0181	0.2524	9	UK
7080	8	m	1963	0.0173	0.2697	8	UK
7086	9	f	1963	0.0162	0.2859	4	IRL
7594	10	m	1965	0.0153	0.3012	7	UK
11730	11	m	1974	0.0144	0.3156	15	UK
9840	12	f	1971	0.0142	0.3298	4	US to UK
9861	13	f	1971	0.0141	0.3439	5	UK
12096	14	m	1974	0.0130	0.3569	6	UK
9103	15	f	1970	0.0117	0.3686	2	UK
8153	16	m	1967	0.0116	0.3802	9	US
8382	17	f	1968	0.0116	0.3918	10	US
6533	18	f	1958	0.0108	0.4026	6	UK
6544	19	m	1958	0.0103	0.4129	5	UK
8420	20	m	1968	0.0100	0.4229	8	Sweden

Table 6.26: Affected population results for PSS. Reading is analogous to table 6.16.

6.4.5 Pedigree Charts for PSS

6.4.5.1 Calculated Ancestors

While the results for the first three causes of death were not particularly encouraging, the PSS data comparisons showed enough promise to put the relations within this population into a pedigree chart. This resulted in figure 6.13 below:

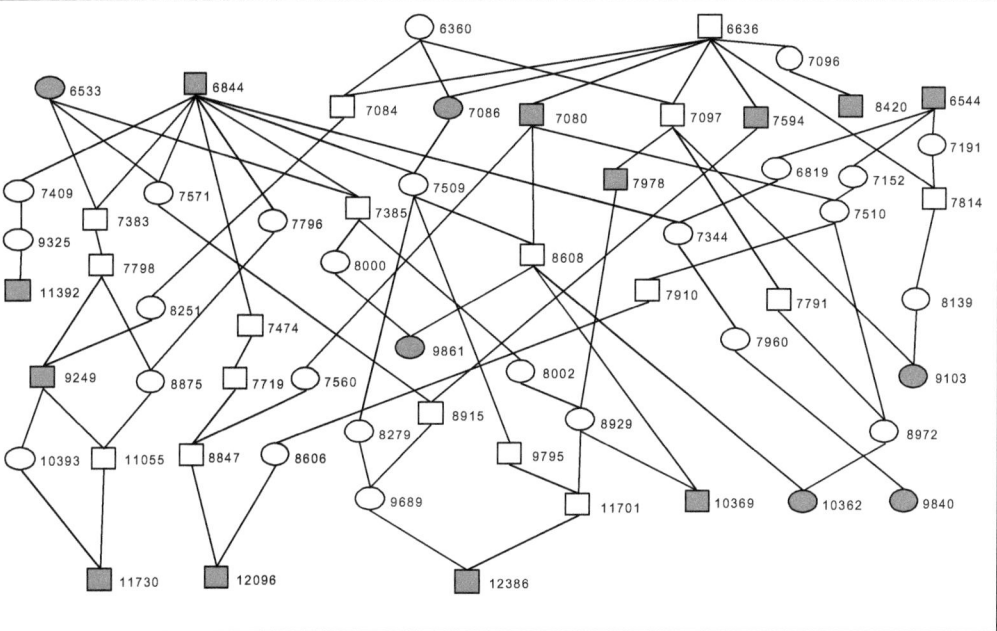

Fig. 6.13*: Pedigree chart of main ancestors of PSS cases (chapter 6.4.4.2). Dogs mentioned in table 6.26 are marked grey.*

Note that individuals 8153 and 8382 have been omitted from this graph. 8153 is a great-grandson of 6360, while 8382 would have to be tracked back behind 5838 to find common ancestors with the population in this graph. Also note that 11'392 is the only individual to appear in the results for both the reference and the affected population.

Given the mode of inheritance (see chapter 3.2.3), the results of this analysis give way to several possible interpretations, which will be investigated further in the following chapters.

6.4.5.2 Dog 6844

Given that dog 6844 explains 6.1% of the genetic variability of all PSS cases, it is obvious that its role in the graph should be analysed. This is done in figure 6.14 below.

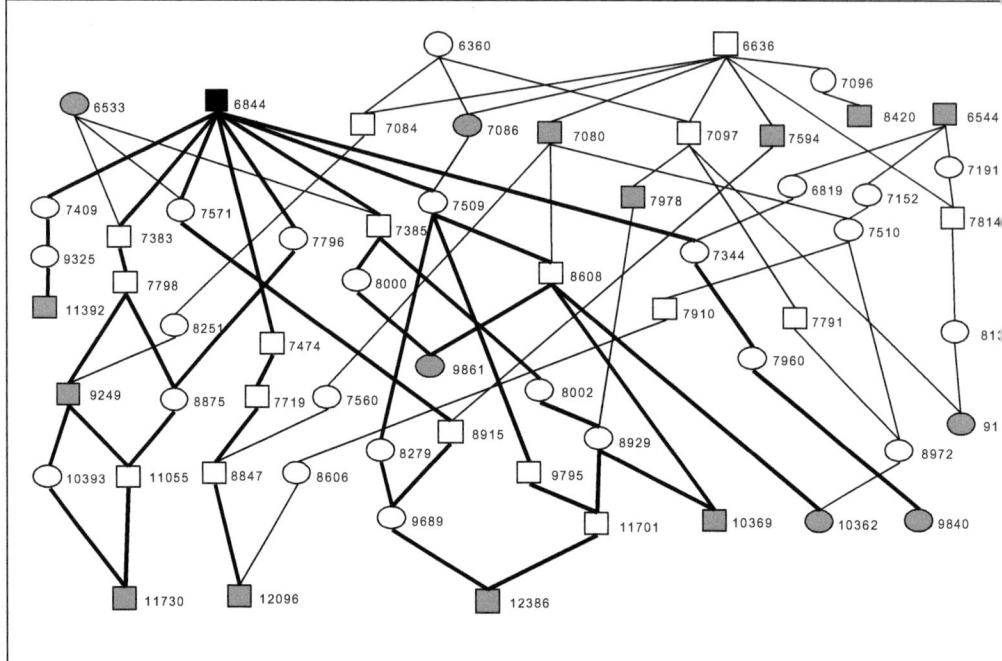

Fig. 6.14: Direct descendants of dog 6844

Figure 6.14 shows that dog 6844 is directly related to all but one important PSS ancestors in the lower half of the pedigree chart, but does in itself not explain the important ancestors in the upper right area of the chart (also see figure 6.16). Within the population marked grey, four double-ups on this individual can be found.

6.4.5.3 Bitch 6360

Despite of not being listed in table 6.26, bitch 6360 (born 1957, UK) was also identified as a relatively important ancestors of the dogs identified through ancestor analysis. Figure 6.15 shows how this individual is related to the other dogs.

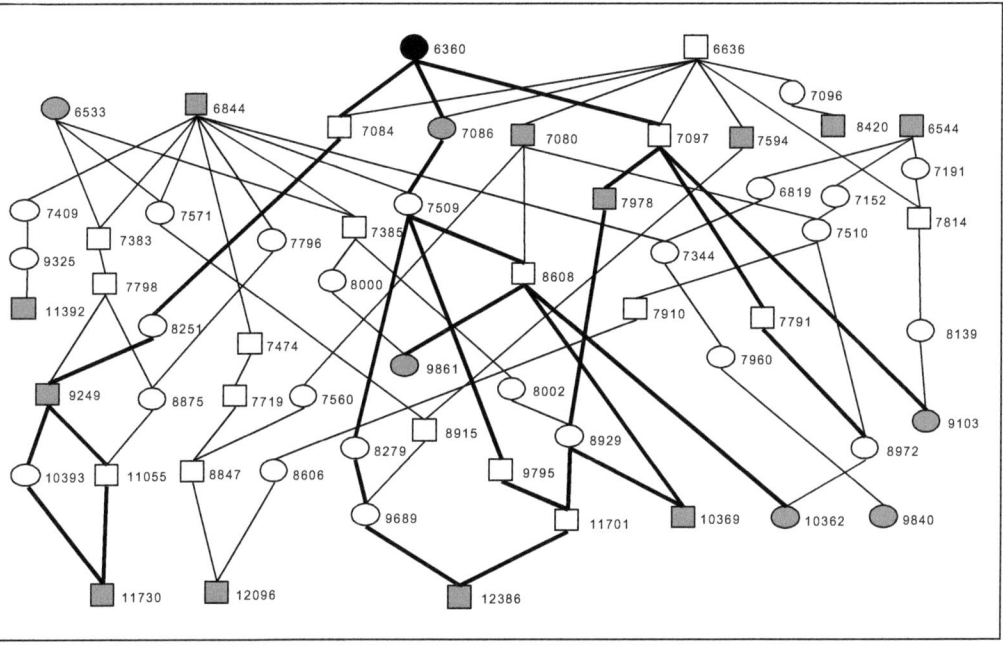

Fig. 6.15: Direct descendants of bitch 6360

This illustration shows that bitch 6360 is also directly related to all but two ancestors in the lower pedigree chart part, but does little to explain the ancestors in the upper row. Within the population marked grey, four double-ups on this individual can be found.

6.4.5.4 Dog 6636

Dog 6636 (born 1959, UK) was also identified as an ancestor of many of the identified important ancestors. His direct descendants are given in figure 6.16 below.

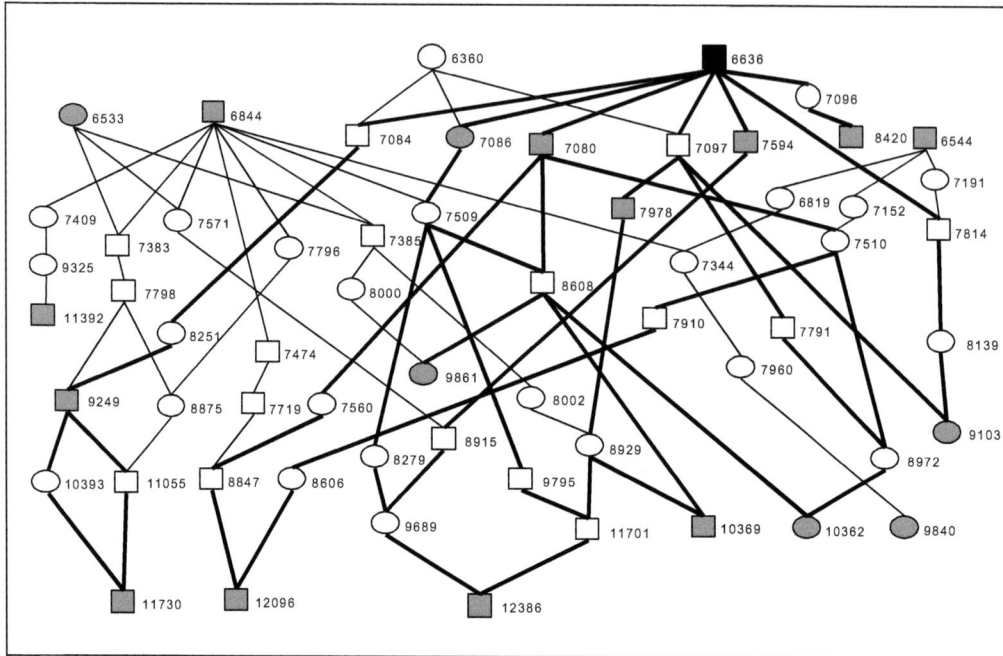

Fig. 6.16*: Direct descendants of dog 6636*

Figure 6.16 shows that in addition to explaining all but one of the important ancestors in the lower pedigree chart, dog 6636 also has direct relations to 5 out of 8 dogs in the top row of the chart. Within the population marked grey, six double-ups in this individual can be found.

6.4.5.5 Ancestors

Given these results, it was decided to also investigate the genetic relations of the ancestors of the individuals marked grey in the upper half of figure 6.16. In order to find a common ancestor of all these individuals, it is necessary to go back to dog 5838 – the same individual that explains 26.02% of genetic variability in the overall database (see table 6.17). Outside of this, dog 6261 (born 1955, UK) and bitch 6026 (1953, UK) might also be of interest due to their additional connection to ancestors 6544 as well as 8420.

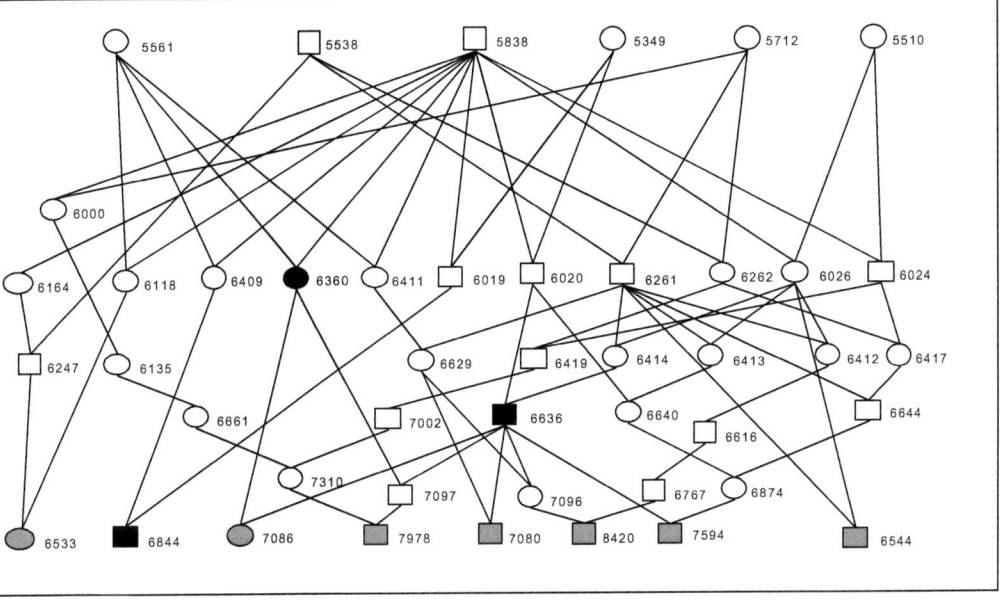

Fig. 6.17: Genetic relations of the aforementioned three dogs (marked black). Additional important ancestors of the population affected with PSS found in this study are marked grey (see table 6.26)

Figure 6.17 also clearly illustrates the genetic bottleneck that occurred with dog 5838, which can be found behind all Irish Wolfhounds alive today. However, the amount of early double-ups done on this dog, as well as the fact that he does not appear on the important ancestor list of affected individuals over 10 generations (see tables 6.25 and 6.26) makes it unlikely that he was a PSS carrier.

7 Discussion

7.1 Lifespan

7.1.1 Lifespan in Large Dogs in General

Several studies have established that large dogs tend to die at a younger age than do smaller ones (Comfort 1960; Deeb and Wolf 1994; Li, Deeb et al. 1996; Patronek, Waters et al. 1997; Michell 1999; Galis, Van Der Sluijs et al. 2006; Greer, Canterberry et al. 2006). This is opposed to the usual biological fact that across the species spectrum, large animals tend to have longer lifespans than do smaller ones.

There is some controversy as to the mechanisms involved; however, the most common current theory is that rapid cell proliferation during the growth phase leads to the accumulation of oxidative DNA damage ("oxidative burst" due to free radicals) early in life. This damage is thought to remain latent for some time, but eventually results in an earlier onset of aging and degenerative disease as well as increased rates of certain cancers. This theory is supported by the finding that adult giant breed dog cells have a lower proliferative capacity than those of other breeds (Li, Deeb et al. 1996), that large dogs tend to develop non-hereditary cataracts (thought to be due to accumulated oxidative damage) at an earlier age than small dogs (Williams, Heath et al. 2004), as well as the finding that dogs fed an energetically restricted diet tend to live longer than dogs fed a regular diet (Kealy, Lawler et al. 2002; Lawler, Evans et al. 2005)

While this mechanism may explain the earlier onset of aging and degenerative disease as well as the earlier outbreak and/or the increased incidence of certain cancer forms in large breeds, it is independent from deaths due to other hereditary diseases and those due to hereditary cancer predispositions.

7.1.2 Significance of Right Censored Data

The influence of right censored data on the measured life expectancy was detected in several previously published studies on canine lifespan. While appropriate statistical methods are often used in human medicine to correct this problem, a literature search showed that this is not the case in the veterinary literature, where lifespan data are routinely derived from death data (Urfer 2008).

In the case of Irish Wolfhounds, it could be shown that previously published lifespan estimates (Bernardi 1986; Prokopenko 1998) had included right censored data and thus underestimated overall life expectancy. While it is clear that such erroneous conclusions need to be pointed out, the author is aware that these finding are also a potential cause for complacency. Therefore, it needs to be pointed out that **even after the correction of right censored data, the results of these studies still make it abundantly clear that the Irish Wolfhound as a breed has a generally poor life expectancy, and that every possible effort should be taken to improve the present situation.**

It was shown that explaining the nature of Cohort Bias through right censored data is not trivial (Urfer and Steiger 2006), but the general problem of right censored data in veterinary lifespan studies goes beyond the scope of this book. For more information on the topic, consult Urfer (2008), which has been included in the appendix of this study.

7.1.3 Differences in Previous Studies' Results

When comparing lifespan calculated from the data of the previously published studies, highly significant differences can be observed between the North American (Bernardi 1986; Prokopenko 1998) and the Anglo-Irish dogs (Murphy 1991), the latter living on average 1.4 years longer than their North American counterparts.

There are several potential interpretations of these differences. Obviously, it is possible that Irish Wolfhounds in Ireland and Great Britain have a higher life expectancy than Irish Wolfhounds in North America. Although the populations are genetically close (see chapter 6.3), the relative isolation due to quarantine laws that existed in Ireland and the UK during the study period may have favoured different developments in this population. The importance of country class in the General Linear Model used for the author's data may also be indicative of this hypothesis.

The distribution of birth cohorts in the two datasets varies: While Bernardi's and Prokopenko's data only contain 6.27% of dogs born before 1965, Murphy (1991) contains 14.04% of such dogs. Since it could be shown in the present study that Irish Wolfhounds lived longer in the 1960s than they did more recently, this may also have had an influence on these differences.

It is also possible that Murphy (1991) was more influenced by submitter's bias (see chapter 3.1.1.1) than were Bernardi (1986) and Prokopenko (1998): The former drew its data almost exclusively from breeders, who may have been more motivated to submit older dogs than to submit those that died young. On the other hand, the North American studies also included significant amounts of data contributed by pet owners, who may have had fewer interests in promoting a particular kennel or family.

These same demographics could also have contributed to the measured lifespan through another mechanism: It could be assumed that people running a breeding kennel may be more educated in veterinary medicine than the average dog owner, which may have lead to an increase in life expectancy in their dogs.

7.1.4 Gender and Castration Effects

The data used in this study unanimously suggest that female Irish Wolfhounds on average have a longer lifespan than do males (chapters 5.1.5, 5.2.1.3 and 6.2.4). While little data have been published about gender effects on lifespan in dogs, this mirrors the situation in humans. It is possible that the shorter life expectancy in males may also be mediated through their larger size to a certain extent.

A gender predisposition of male Irish Wolfhounds to Dilatative Cardiomyopathy has been described in numerous studies (see chapter 3.3.2) and was also reproduced in the study at hand (see chapters 5.1.5 and 6.2.4), thus further supporting the hypothesis that a sex predisposition for this disease exists in the breed.

The predisposition of female Irish Wolfhounds to death by cancers other than Osteosarcoma has not been described in the literature beforehand. However, the findings of the study at hand are identical to those derived from the data of Bernardi (1986) and Prokopenko (1998) as described in chapters 5.1.5 and 6.2.4, providing considerable support for this hypothesis. Unfortunately, no sufficient data on which types of cancer account for this phenomenon were available.

Castration showed a considerable lifespan benefit in female Irish Wolfhounds in this study, which is consistent with what is generally accepted in the literature. In male Irish Wolfhounds, however, a non-significant decrease in life expectancy, as well as a significant increase in Osteosarcoma risk was found in castrated animals. This mirrors findings in other studies, where castration has been associated with an increase in osteosarcoma risk (Ru, Terracini et al. 1998; Cooley, Beranek et al. 2002). However, no such risk increase was found in castrated female Irish Wolfhounds in the study at hand as opposed to the two quoted studies.

It is possible that the increase in OS risk in castrated males may be partially mediated through a longer growth period in males that underwent early castration. However, other hormone-mediated effects are likely to also play a role in this context. Given that neither a lifespan benefit nor a decrease in any particular cause of death associated with male castration could be demonstrated in the study at hand, it seems advisable not to routinely subject male Irish Wolfhounds to the procedure. If the owner insists on the operation, it should at least be postponed until after the end of the animal's growth period.

7.1.5 Development of Lifespan Over Time

As shown in chapter 6.2.6, there was a highly significant diminution of life expectancy in dogs born since the 1960s. Furthermore, although lifespan data from before this period are scarce in the database used for this study, other results (Comfort 1956) suggest that there seems to be a phase of increasing lifespan, then a point when a maximal lifespan was reached in dogs born in the 1960s, followed by a period where it dropped again, to the point where life expectancy of Irish Wolfhounds born 1990-1993 was decreased by roughly 1½ years as compared to their ancestors born during the 1960s.

The reasons for this development are difficult to ascertain. Obviously, the increasing possibilities of canine veterinary health care that became available in the years following 1960 are a possible candidate to explain the increase in lifespan during this period – the widespread introduction of effective veterinary vaccination programs in this decade in particular has probably played a key role, as may be the case with the wider availability of antibiotic and antiparasitic drugs. However, this does not explain why lifespan subsequently started to drop again despite the fact that the quality of available veterinary care continued to increase.

Natural selection – "survival of the fittest" – may have influenced the observed development: Back when veterinary care was more limited in its possibilities, Irish Wolfhounds were subject to selection by their natural fitness and vigour. Even in the absence of conscious selection for health and vigour traits, it was less common for weaker individuals to be used for breeding, since they were eliminated from the gene pool at an earlier age; most probably due to infectious diseases. This may have contributed to a selection for vigour as well as continuous purging phenomena (see chapter 7.2.2.3) in the breeding population, which could then realise its full genetic potential once deaths due to infectious diseases were decreased due to the more widespread availability of vaccines and antibiotics. However, since the previously accumulated fitness no longer determined a dog's use in reproduction after the aforementioned improvements in veterinary care, selection pressure for fitness and vigour traits as well as allele purging were markedly decreased. Consequently, dogs with weaker fitness traits were and are given more influence on the gene pool, contributing to the measured decrease in mean lifespan.

Similarly, it is likely that the exponential increase in the population after 1960 also had an influence on the reduction of selection pressure on the breeding population, which might also have contributed to the decrease in lifespan.

Considering that conscious selection for breeding in purebred dogs – including Irish Wolfhounds – is usually influenced by dog show results, it is possible that one or several of the post-1960s popular sires were passing such low-vigour and/or hereditary disease traits to their progeny in addition to the general tendency towards a decrease of selection pressure for vigour. Given the small genetic base of the breed, their traits could subsequently have become widespread throughout the population ("Founder Effect"). Dog 1 (and possibly 2) in chapter 6.2.5 is a possible candidate for such a mechanism. While he does not appear in the PEDIG 10-generation ancestor analyses that were performed during this study due to the birth cohorts chosen (1965-2005), he does play an important role in the genetic makeup of the modern population and, as a direct ancestor of several other more recent popular sires, can be found in the pedigree of the majority of Irish Wolfhounds alive today.

The lack of deaths by osteosarcoma in an earlier sample (Comfort 1956) may be in favour of the hypothesis that disease distribution in the breed has changed over time, with improved veterinary care as well as the individual contributions of some popular sires being probable causes as explained above. However, our own data did not include a sufficient number of deaths with known causes to accurately test this hypothesis.

Another hypothesis is that there could be one or several distinct genetic "longevity" vs. "short lifespan" traits that are independent from other genetic predispositions to specific causes of death. This could explain why a previous study (Bernardi 1986) found no increase in life expectancy after the most common causes of death were excluded (see chapter 3.1.3.1). However, if this were the case, one would expect to not only find sires that distinctly pass on a low life expectancy to their progeny, but also some sires that pass on an increased one ("producers of longevity"). While there are some such dogs in the results found in chapter 6.2.5, differences amongst them are not significant. Although this in itself does not exclude the possibility of distinct "longevity" and "short lifespan" genes, it makes it likely that such "longevity" genes would be recessive in nature and their effects become overridden by both hereditary diseases and "short lifespan" traits. This would in principle also be compatible with the decreased lifespan in combination with a decrease in short-term inbreeding coefficients.

In view of the finding that female castration improves life expectancy significantly, whereas male castration, while increasing osteosarcoma risk, does not seem to reduce lifespan significantly, and assuming that both male and female castration have become more common during the past 30 years, it is unlikely that the practice has had an influence on the overall decrease in lifespan – on the contrary, female castration at least can be expected to have counteracted the tendency to a certain degree. The fact that average lifespan still decreased considerably despite the increasing incidence of female castration in the breed is thus another reason for concern regarding its current state of health.

A general phenomenon that can be observed since the 1960s is the tendency of dog breeding to change from a state in which a few large kennels existing over long periods of time and having a comparably large number of breeding stock on which to base their selection are replaced by many smaller kennels that only keep a small number of dogs and exist during a more limited amount of time. Such smaller kennels often select their breeding stock based on emotional considerations rather than objective breeding value in both health and conformation, and having fewer bitches available implies an additional loss of possible breeding options and, consequently, a decrease in selection pressure (Sommerfeld-Stur 2005).

Finally, it is not impossible (though highly improbable by the findings of the present study) that the increase in lifespan seen in the 1960s could be due to the outcross to dog 5838, leading to a temporary decrease in the overall level of inbreeding in the Anglo-Irish population. While the findings of this study concerning the lack of inbreeding influence on life expectancy (see chapters 6.2.3 and 6.2.7) do not support this hypothesis, and while one would not expect a similar increase and decrease in lifespan to be seen in North American Dogs from the same period, it is impossible to entirely exclude the possibility.

7.2 Population Genetics

7.2.1 Population History and Genetic Bottleneck Phenomena

While the existence of large sighthound-like wolf-hunting dogs from Ireland is reported time and again throughout recorded history (Symmachus 393; Graham 1885; Walker 1896; Hogan 1897; Gardner 1931; DeQuoy 1971; DeQuoy 1973; Miller 1988; Maison 1990; DeQuoy 1991; DeQuoy, Castillo et al. 1993; McBryde 1998; Thomasson 1999; Doyle 2002), the history of modern Irish Wolfhounds as studied in this thesis starts in the 1860s, when Captain George Augustus Graham defined the modern breed standard and started a controlled breeding program with the goal of recreating the breed that was, by then, almost extinct. To achieve this goal, he bred dogs that were believed to be related to the original Irish Wolfhound to other breeds of great size, such as Scottish Deerhounds, Great Danes and a variety of other dogs. Consult the above references for more detailed descriptions of the exact modus operandi.

Based on the present data, the population history of modern Irish Wolfhounds can be roughly divided into the following phases:

Time Period	Phase	N°
ca. 1860-1890	Start of modern Irish Wolfhound breeding by Capt. Graham and associates. **First genetic bottleneck**.	1
ca. 1890-1914	Consolidation period; occasional further outcrossing. Increase of population size.	2
1914- ca. 1920	World War I: decrease of population size; inbreeding peak. **Second genetic bottleneck**.	3
ca. 1920-1939	Economic prosperity; population size increases even throughout the Great Depression	4
1939-1952	World War II: population size greatly reduced, strong inbreeding on dog 4732 in the UK and IRL. **Third genetic bottleneck**.	
1952	Import of dog 5838 from the USA to the UK; short decrease of inbreeding due to widespread use of this individual.	5
since 1952	Dog 5838 becomes widespread throughout all Irish Wolfhound pedigrees. **Fourth genetic bottleneck**.	
since 1965	Exponential increase of population size masks previous inbreeding in Wright's Inbreeding Coefficients.	6

Table 7.1: Phases of the history of the modern Irish Wolfhound population. The N° column refers to Fig. 7.1 below.

As shown in chapter 6.3.2, the last two genetic bottlenecks have the most influence on the population born 1965-2005. Of course, it should be kept in mind that the dogs shown to be the most important ancestors of this population are still subject to the genetic consequences of the previous two bottlenecks

Figure 7.1 gives a typical example of the complete pedigree of an Irish Wolfhound born in 2000. Every ancestor is listed only once and connected to all individuals in its first-generation progeny. The broadness of the genogram thus gives an impression of the effective breeding population size at a given time.

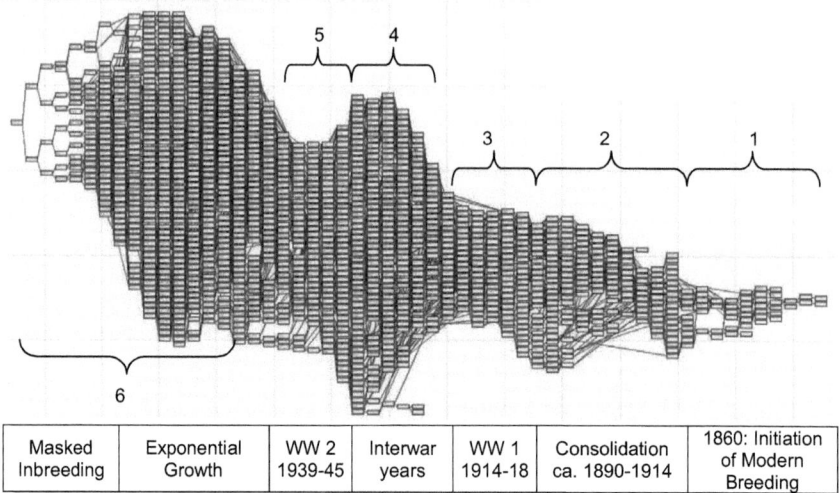

Fig. 7.1: *Typical genogram of an Irish Wolfhound born in 2000 (field in the far left), illustrating the occurrence of several genetic bottlenecks during the history of the population. The numbers in the figure refer to the occurrences described in table 7.1 above. Compare this graph to fig. 6.3 and 6.4*

Note that the third and fourth genetic bottleneck do not appear as separate occurrences in this graph due to their closeness in time. The studied individual is subject to an average level of inbreeding (COI(5)=0.0078; COI(10)=0.1120; COI(20)=0.2707; Meuwissen's Inbreeding Coefficient = 0.3470).

7.2.2 Inbreeding and Lifespan

7.2.2.1 Mechanisms of Inbreeding Depression

Inbreeding depression cannot occur if gene effects are purely additive – some degree of dominance and/or epistatic interaction between genes is necessary. Currently, there are two main theories on the genetic mechanisms underlying inbreeding depression: The partial dominance model and the overdominance model (Charlesworth and Charlesworth 1987).

The partial dominance model of inbreeding depression postulates that inbreeding depression is caused by the accumulation of recessive deleterious alleles that can occur as the degree of homozygosis increases. This accumulation of recessive deleterious alleles ("genetic load") that are normally masked by dominance effects in the heterozygous form results in a loss of fitness in the inbred population, which can be expected to be proportional to the degree of deleteriousness in the relevant alleles.

On the other hand, the overdominance model postulates that inbreeding depression is not merely caused by the accumulation of recessive deleterious alleles, but rather results from a decrease in heterozygosis itself. Heterozygous individuals are thought to have inherently higher fitness values ("heterosis") than homozygous ones in this model, which may be influenced by epistatic gene effects.

Current research points to inbreeding depression being mainly due to partial dominance phenomena, although some contribution by overdominance cannot be ruled out (Charlesworth and Charlesworth 1987; Lacy and Ballou 1998; Crnokrak and Barrett 2002; Ayroles, Hughes et al. 2009).

7.2.2.2 Lack of Inbreeding Depression in Other Models

Examples for heavily inbred mammal populations with little to no apparent inbreeding depression are numerous and include, amongst others, inbred strains of laboratory mice and rats, captive golden hamsters (*Mesocricetus auratus*), a subspecies of *Peromyscus polionotus* (Lacy, Alaks et al. 1996; Lacy and Ballou 1998), Chillingham wild cattle (Visscher, Smith et al. 2001), captive Speke's Gazelles (Templeton and Read 1984), and Icelandic horses (Sommerfeld-Stur, personal communication). The Kromfohrländer dog is also a likely candidate due to its genetic history (Urfer and Eberli, unpublished data; see chapter 7.2.3). Apart from mammals, such populations have also been described in plants and non-mammalian animals (Thornhill 1993).

When enumerating such examples, however, it should be kept in mind that they do not in themselves challenge the fact that inbreeding depression is a very real phenomenon in the majority of mammals, and that an apparent lack found in one population should always be considered in view of the population's genetic history, as well as its environment (Hedrick and Kalinowski 2000). Extrapolating the findings of the study at hand to other populations may therefore be inappropriate.

7.2.2.3 Allele Purging

"Purging the genetic load" refers to a phenomenon that can occur if inbreeding depression is mainly due to the partial dominance mechanism: During phases of continuous inbreeding, individuals that are homozygous for deleterious alleles have reduced fitness and consequently produce fewer offspring, leading to a decrease and/or eventual elimination of such deleterious alleles from the population (Crnokrak and Barrett 2002).

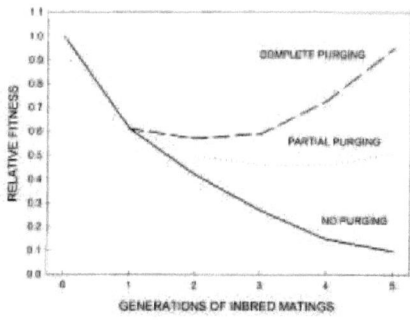

Fig. 7.2: Three possible scenarios for purging of the genetic load. No purging: fitness of inbred lines continues to decrease linearly with successive generations of inbreeding. Partial purging: inbred line fitness decreases initially, then rebounds to approximately 50% of outbred level. Complete purging: after an initial drop, inbred lines recover fitness values to levels comparable to original level. Graph taken from Crokrak and Barrett (2002), modified after Lacy and Ballou (1998)

In this model, the degree of purging to be expected would be influenced by the degree of deleteriousness in the alleles considered: An allele that is only mildly deleterious can be expected to undergo only limited amounts of purging during a phase of inbreeding, while a highly deleterious allele would be more likely to be completely eliminated.

7.2.2.4 Bottleneck Scenarios

A genetic bottleneck occurs when a small number of founders are selected out of the population to create the new population. This can be expected to change the overall allele frequency, causing the alleles the founders were carrying to become widespread throughout the new population. The increase in inbreeding and thus homozygosis can be expected to lead to purging phenomena in some cases, making a recovery of fitness possible if the deleterious alleles are subject to selection (Fowler and Whitlock 1999; Kirkpatrick and Jarne 2000).

It has been demonstrated that a bottleneck can be expected to reduce susceptibility to inbreeding depression in a population, since it reduces the genetic variation, thus leading to a smaller difference in fitness between offspring from random matings and offspring from matings between relatives. However, it will at the same time increase the genetic load, since the effects of homozygous deleterious alleles can be expected to be greater than the positive effect from loci where a deleterious allele is lost. This mechanism will result in an increase in inbreeding depression immediately after the bottleneck as compared to the pre-bottleneck state; the increase being most substantial when the bottleneck is extreme and the mutations are highly recessive. This will be followed by a recovery period during which purging of the genetic load takes place, the intensity of which is dependent on the degree of recessivity of the allele, the decrease in fitness it entails, the average DNA mutation rate, and the rate of population growth after the bottleneck. It will continue for as long as the purging effects continue to be a more important factor than the accumulation of new mutations in the gene pool (Kirkpatrick and Jarne 2000).

It has been calculated that inbreeding depression will continue to decline in the following generations for as long as the following criteria are met:

$$h < \frac{N}{5N-s}$$

Where h is the coefficient of dominance of the mutated allele, N is the number of founders in the bottleneck, and s is the selection coefficient, i.e. the measure of the degree by which biological fitness is diminished by the mutation. This inequation shows that at least some purging can be expected to occur for all mutants that are more recessive than approximately 0.2 (Kirkpatrick and Jarne 2000).

In the same article, it has also been demonstrated that the decrease in inbreeding effects after a genetic bottleneck are most marked in case of a slow rather than a fast population growth after the bottleneck, caused by the more important effects of post-bottleneck genetic drift.

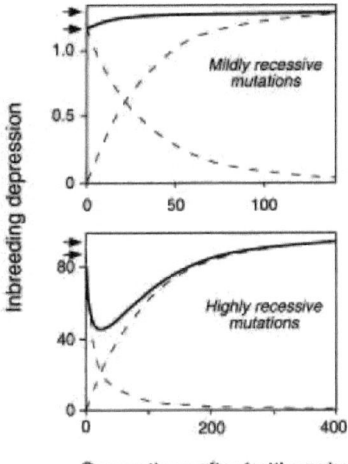

Fig. 7.3: Recovery of inbreeding depression contributed by a single locus following a bottleneck of size 5 as a function of time (in generations). Values of the depression have been multiplied by 10^6. Upper panel, mildly recessive mutation with $h=0.3$ and $s=0.1$. Lower panel, highly recessive lethal with $h=0.01$ and $s=1.0$. For both panels, $\mu=10^{-6}$ (μ=allelic mutation rate). Arrows on the left of each panel indicate the inbreeding depression at equilibrium (upper arrow) and immediately following the bottleneck (lower arrow).

The ascending dashed curves show the contributions from loci that lose the deleterious allele during the bottleneck, and the declining curves the contributions from loci where the bottleneck causes the mutant frequency to increase. Graph taken from Kirkpatrick and Jarne (2000).

However, Kirkpatrick and Jarne (2000) also showed that the genetic load can be expected to fall below baseline some generations after a genetic bottleneck, provided that population growth is slow and the deleterious alleles are highly recessive.

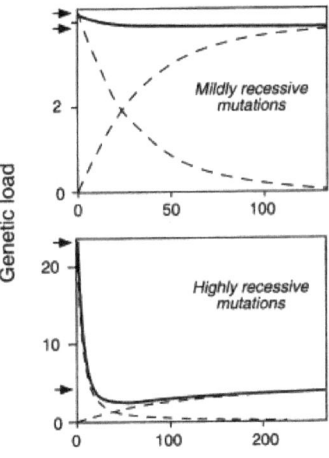

Fig.7.4: Recovery of the genetic load contributed by a single locus following a bottleneck of size 5 as a function of time (in generations). Values of the load have been multiplied by 10^6. Upper panel, mildly recessive mutation with $h=0.3$ and $s=0.1$. Lower panel, highly recessive lethal with $h=0.01$ and $s=1.0$. For both panels, $\mu=10^{-6}$ (μ=allelic mutation rate). Arrows on the left of each panel indicate the load at equilibrium (lower arrow) and immediately following the bottleneck (upper arrow). The ascending dashed curves show the contributions from loci that lose the deleterious allele during the bottleneck, and the declining curves the contributions from loci where the bottleneck causes the mutant frequency to increase. Graph taken from Kirkpatrick and Jarne (2000).

It must also be kept in mind that whenever a population goes through a genetic bottleneck, substantial random selection effects can be expected to happen. Thus, susceptibility to inbreeding depression in populations following a genetic bottleneck can be expected to also be influenced by random founder effects (Fowler and Whitlock 1999).

7.2.2.5 Present Study

No significant effects of inbreeding on lifespan were detected in any of the analyses performed during this study. Also, while on first view, there seems to be an apparent correlation between the increase of Meuwissen's inbreeding coefficient and the decreasing lifespan in the late 1960s (see Fig. 6.4 and 6.11, as well as table 6.13), the statistical analyses presented in chapters 6.2.3 and 6.2.7 make it unlikely that this correlation is causal.

Apart from a decrease in lifespan, other possible effects of inbreeding have been described in the veterinary literature. This notably includes decreased fertility parameters, such as the percentage of fertile matings, litter size, and peripartal mortality rate (Peyer 1997). Their importance in Irish Wolfhounds could not be assessed in the present study due to incomplete data on complete litters and no data on failed matings in the database. However, a new study on inbreeding and fertility in Irish Wolfhounds in Sweden by the author of the study at hand found no such effect in the studied population (Urfer 2009). Its text is reproduced in the appendix.

While the apparent lack of inbreeding depression in this study might be surprising or even confusing at first glance, it may be explained through the genetic history of the modern Irish Wolfhound population. Given that the breed is highly inbred and went through several genetic bottlenecks during its modern history, allele purging phenomena and other bottleneck effects can be expected to have taken place somewhere in the past (see chapters 7.2.2.2 to 7.2.2.4 above). This would imply that inbreeding depression caused by the accumulation of recessive deleterious alleles has been eliminated in the breed as far as lifespan is concerned.

Alternatively, it is also possible that Irish Wolfhounds have reached a very high level of homozygosity long ago, to a point where further inbreeding is unlikely to further increase its possible detrimental effects. This hypothesis was already favoured by Comfort (1956) (see chapter 3.1.2.1). However, given that we do not have access to a pre-bottleneck Irish Wolfhound population with which to compare inbreeding depression, the distinction between these two hypotheses is of academic interest at best.

Furthermore, it could be that improved housing conditions counteract detrimental effects of inbreeding depression (Kalinowski, Hedrick et al. 2000). However, this is not consistent with the decrease in lifespan in Irish Wolfhounds that occurred after the introduction of modern veterinary medicine.

Based on the above models, it could also be asked whether the rapid population growth in Irish Wolfhounds since 1965 has contributed to the observed decrease in lifespan due to the accumulation of new deleterious alleles. If this were the case, however, we would expect to find an influence of inbreeding coefficients over a short number of generations, which was not the case (see chapter 6.2.3). While this does not exclude the possibility that such a development could take place in the future, it should also be kept in mind that the accumulation of such mutations takes a very long time.

Given the genetic history of the breed as well as the findings of the study at hand, it seems likely that further inbreeding in Irish Wolfhounds will not per se result in a decrease in lifespan in the foreseeable future.

7.2.3 Ancestor Analysis

It could be shown that Irish Wolfhounds alive today are highly inbred and that this fact tends to be masked in more recent pedigrees due to the exponential population growth that has occurred since the 1960s. The extreme importance of very few ancestors is not uncommon in purebred dogs, but these bottlenecks tend to date from a more distant past in most modern dog breeds. A notable exception is the Kromfohrländer dog, which can be tracked back completely to three individuals, two dating from the years immediately following WW2 and the third born in 1957 (Urfer and Eberli, unpublished data).

The genetic bottlenecks in Irish Wolfhounds during WW1 and WW2 can be explained by a combination of geographical and political factors: First, the Irish Wolfhound breeding population was small and geographically limited to the UK, Ireland and North America during these times. While their relative indemnity from direct acts of war prevented a total extinction in the way it occurred in continental Europe, keeping significant numbers of large dogs was extremely difficult even in these countries due to widespread food rationing. Thus, the breeding population strongly decreased in numbers during these times of war.

While one could argue that there were two separate breeding populations in the British Isles and North America (even though they shared the same origins), these were mixed following both WW1 (dog 3132 et al.) and WW2 (dog 5838 et al.), and exchanges of breeding stock across the Atlantic can be observed repeatedly.

Given this population history, it is no surprise to find that the last two genetic bottlenecks around WW2 exercise the strongest influence on the analysed population, even when analysing the population back to its origins in the mid-19th century. The relatively narrow timeframe of the twenty most important ancestors of the population born 1965-2005 is also indicative of this fact.

7.2.4 Diseases Presumed Hereditary

The results of ancestor analysis for diseases presumed hereditary are somewhat difficult to interpret. Given that a sufficient amount of health data of complete litters was unavailable in the database used for this study, it is impossible to determine an exact mode of inheritance using our approach; however, it is possible to identify a present hereditary component without information on the health of whole litters being necessary.

Given the observed genetic bottlenecks throughout population history, it was only logical that no differences in ancestors between affected individuals and their respective reference populations could be observed when calculating all the way back to the origins of our population. Meaningful differences could only be expected by limiting the number of generations considered, which we did by limiting analysis to ten generations.

It is interesting to consider what results this method of analysis would yield for a disease that is caused by mutations that occurred before the last genetic bottleneck. Presumably, no differences would be evident between the affected and the reference populations when calculating further back than the most recent genetic bottleneck. In any case, the method used does not allow us to track any particular mutation farther back than the last genetic bottleneck, and given that reliable health data that can be linked to pedigrees do not exist beyond this point, it is likely that attempts to identify carriers of hereditary diseases that date from before WW2 will remain merely speculative.

7.2.4.1 DCM, OS and GDV

Notable ancestor differences between the affected and reference populations were observed in all three diseases when calculating back 10 generations. However, as is evident in table 9.1 (rendered in the appendix), the ancestor patterns of all three affected populations show remarkable similarities. This could reflect a tendency of dogs with known causes of death to come from similar backgrounds, which could be due to confounding factors in data collection, such as varying willingness amongst breeders of different geographical origin to contribute health data of their dogs.

Another possible explanation is that the apparent genetic similarities in the ancestors of the populations affected with these three diseases may reflect the impact of varying breeding philosophies: Being more tolerant of hereditary problems may be a non-specific trait in some breeders, leading to an increased frequency of several hereditary diseases in their particular families.

The analysis of the reference populations (see chapter 4.5) for these three diseases shows a good overlap with the ancestors of the population born between 1965 and 2005, indicating that the data should be representative of the overall population.

It is also interesting to note that the individual percentual importance of the most important ancestors of the affected populations is lower than it is for the reference populations.

In the case of DCM, the correlation between its frequency and an increase of inbreeding published in a previous study (Broschk 2004) could not be reproduced when analysing the present data (see chapter 6.2.3.2)

7.2.4.2 Portosystemic Shunt

The results of ancestor analysis for PSS show some striking differences from the other three analysed categories, making it likely that a genetic influence was detected in this case. Interestingly, the most important ancestors in the reference population also show some differences from the other reference populations. This can most likely be explained by the circumstance that all but one of the disease cases in the affected population date from 1984 to 2004, whereas the disease cases for the previous three categories show a more even distribution since the mid-1960s.

The only individual to appear in both the affected and the reference populations' ancestors is dog 11392, who can thus be considered an "innocent bystander" by the results of this analysis.

Another interesting observation is that the top twenty 10-generation ancestors of the affected population have significantly more recent years of birth than those of the reference population (P=0.0002, R^2=0.3170, F=17.64; type III SS). This implies a shorter generation interval in the families affected with PSS. While it is possible that the breeders of the Wolfhound families where PSS originated simply had/have the habit of using their dogs for breeding at a younger-than-average age, it could also be that the occurrence of PSS in a family would lead to a number of dogs dying at a relatively young age, increasing the incentive for the breeders to use their dogs for breeding at a younger age due to the fear of otherwise losing them before they could produce offspring.

While the nature of the calculations employed makes it impossible to prove or disprove the published mode of inheritance (van Steenbeek, Leegwater et al. 2009), the results of this study still allow to provide some answers to questions that have been asked about PSS. Notably, the hypothesis that PSS was originally introduced to the UK Irish Wolfhound population from North America can be considered highly unlikely: It would seem that the current problem originated in the UK and was introduced to the population from there.

The results suggest that PSS in Irish Wolfhounds could be caused by a mutation that has occurred after the last genetic bottleneck. However, when considering this hypothesis, several points should be mentioned: For instance, there is some evidence that the closely Wolfhound-related Scottish Deerhound is affected with a type of PSS that is similar to the Wolfhound form (White, Burton et al. 1998), despite the fact that the last reported crosses between these two breeds took place in the 1930s (Anonymous 1922-2005).

If the mutation took place after the last genetic bottleneck, the results presented in chapter 6.4.5 suggest dog 6636 to be the likely original carrier. While it is probable that this individual was indeed a carrier, the structure of the present population makes it impossible to determine whether he spontaneously developed the mutation or inherited it from another ancestor. The question of when and where the original PSS mutation occurred remains thus unanswered and is unlikely to ever be resolved beyond doubt.

As an aside, it should also be noted that individuals 12'386, 10'369, 10'362 and 7080 in table 6.26 were all bred by the same kennel and explain 11.51% of genetic variability in the affected population altogether. While this does not identify this particular kennel as the direct and sole responsible for the entire modern PSS problem, it may nevertheless imply a certain degree of causality.

According to the database, a direct descendant of dog 12'386 (Wright's Relationship Coefficient over 10 generations: 52.24%) has been used at stud at least 41 times between 1993 and 2005. This does not constitute the absolute record in the database (equalised by a male who was also used at stud 41 times between 1972 and 1977); however, it marks the most popular sire of recent times and thus the dog that will probably become the next genetic bottleneck of the breed. Considering the close genetic relations to dog 12'386, and considering that a full sibling of this individual has been used at stud an additional 23 times between 1995 and 2002, this represents a considerable risk of further spreading of the disease throughout the population.

7.3 Ethical Considerations

7.3.1 Introduction

This section is based on the premise that there are two distinct core interests involved in all aspects of dog breeding: canine interests and human interests. While there are interests that are only applicable to particular situations on both sides, many of them can be stated in a more general form. These two interests are overlapping in many cases; however, most of the important ethical issues arise in the situations where they are not. Thus, both should be clearly separated and weighed against each other whenever considering ethical issues.

7.3.1.1 Canine Interests

Canine interests can be divided into individual and collective interests, i.e. interests of the individual dog and collective interests of the whole population, which can also be called interests of the breed.

Individual interests can be summarised under the interest to live in an environment that is appropriate to the dogs' species-specific physiological and behavioural needs, also including their physical health (self-preservation; food, shelter, veterinary medical care, grooming; canine and human social contact and interaction, mental stimulation; adequate exercise etc).

Interests of the population can be summarised under the interest of population preservation and thus the interest to keep disease levels in the population sufficiently low and fertility parameters sufficiently high for natural reproduction to remain possible in an appropriately favourable environment. Given that dog breeds themselves are artificially created entities, the degree to which this applies to a given breed rather than the dog population as a whole can be questioned, rendering this interest overlapping with human interests.

7.3.1.2 Human Interests

Human interests can be divided into breeders' interests, buyers' and owners' interests, and the interests of the general public. Breeders' and owners' interests are overlapping in some aspects, since all breeders are also owners. The points enumerated in the following paragraph can therefore be considered specific to breeders, but do not exclude the existence of interests in breeders that are listed under "owners' interests".

Specific breeders' interests can be summarised under the desire to get emotional gain out of the act of breeding, with potential financial gain only playing a secondary role in most cases (Sommerfeld-Stur 2005). This may include the interest to get a litter out of a specific bitch kept at the kennel, which increases as the number of bitches per kennel decreases; the interest to have dogs that win at dog shows and become champions, the interest of having a stud dog that can be used on other bitches to produce champions and, secondarily, to generate income; and the interest of cultivating a positive self-image (e.g. as an "artist", or in view of one's position in "breed history", or through the impression that one is "improving the breed"). The latter two interests can also result in breeders being secretive with regard to health conditions in their particular family of dogs, which can be an obstacle to efficient health-oriented selection.

Generally spoken, considering a live animal a means of artistic expression similar to a canvas or a piece of clay is a condescending point of view that reduces the animal to a status similar to the one it held in the Cartesian view: essentially an emotionless object that humans have the right to freely manipulate for their own egotistical goals.

The problem of considering "personal experience" to be more meaningful than scientifically established data also forms part of this spectrum: Subjective personal impressions, which are not usually based on a significant number of observations, nor on any statistical evaluation thereof, can be considered superior to objective collection and evaluation of data in such cases, which can also inhibit health-oriented selection. In certain cases, this attitude may also lead to the repudiation of scientific methods and evidence (such as health tests or the use of genetic principles) in favour of subjective opinion, based on "personal experience" as defined above.

Buyers' and owners' interests include acquiring and keeping a dog that conforms to the general standard of the breed in both appearance and personality and thus the continued availability of such dogs; being able to relate emotionally to their dog; having a dog that is generally healthy, lives as long as possible in good health and causes them as few problems as possible during its life. Additional interests may include the need for a dog that stands a chance of doing well at dog shows, lure coursing events or other forms of canine activities, and/or having a dog that is representative of a social status.

While an emotional relation to a dog or a group of dogs can, in itself, be considered something positive, it also carries the risk of assessing and selecting breeding stock through the proverbial "rose-tinted glasses". This in turn represents another mechanism trough which selection pressure on the breed is weakened, making the owner's motivation to breed rather than the objective genetic quality of the dog the main base for selection (Sommerfeld-Stur 2005).

The interests of the general public are often expressed in a political motivation to ensure animal welfare, which can be directed against the breeding of dogs perceived to be "Qualzucht". This German-language expression is difficult to translate into English, but can be summarised under the concept that certain physical, physiological and/or psychical attributes that are sought for in the breed standard are a cause of health problems and/or suffering for the animal. In the case of Irish Wolfhounds, the low lifespan as well as certain size-associated health problems (notably osteosarcoma and the diseases of the OC/OCD spectrum) are sometimes perceived as criteria to warrant their inclusion in such a category (Peyer 1997).

The interests of the general public also include the motivation to omit harm being done to humans through accidents involving aggressive dogs. Recently, legislations to ban the breeding and import of dog breeds considered dangerous have been adopted under various national jurisdictions. While Irish Wolfhounds have not been included in such lists to-date, their mere size could potentially result in the breed becoming a target for such legislation.

7.3.2 Decreased Lifespan

The ethical implications of a decreased lifespan are not evident at first glance. Although intuitively, it would seem correct that an overall decrease in lifespan in a breed of dog is an ethical problem in breeding, it could be argued that as long as the decrease is not accompanied by an increase in suffering, and given that animals lack an understanding of the concept of death, a decrease in lifespan could be considered acceptable.

For example, the preliminary death out of entirely human interests is usually considered acceptable in food animals that are slaughtered for human consumption as long as their associated suffering is minimised. Hence, it could be argued that a decrease in lifespan that is associated with other human interests (such as show wins etc. as enumerated in the previous chapter) can also be acceptable.

Of course, one difference is that in the case of slaughtering, preliminary death is arbitrarily and deliberately inflicted on the animal, whereas it is merely implicitly accepted as a likely consequence in the case of certain Irish Wolfhound breeding practices. It could also be argued that the human interest of satisfying personal vanity should be considered less important than the primary need for food in an omnivorous mammal. Whether one way of dying should be considered less "natural" than the other, however, could be a subject of considerable debate.

Apart from the utilitarian point of view, the question of animal suffering still plays an important role, for it is evident that many of the important causes of death in Irish Wolfhounds, as well as the diseases of the OC/OCD spectrum, are accompanied by some degree of suffering. From this point of view, it can be argued that six months of affliction by a painful disease represent a higher percentage of overall lifespan in a dog that dies at six years of age than in one that dies at twelve. A shortened lifespan, while not a primary cause of suffering, can thus be considered a cause of a relative increase in suffering throughout life.

But even apart from the pathocentric point of view, the decrease in lifespan due to breeding practices represents an ethical problem in itself. For example, few would agree that creating a hypothetical breed of dog with a lifespan of two years followed by painless death would be ethically acceptable. Even though dogs presumably lack an understanding of the concept of death, they, like any other living creature, are governed by a powerful instinct of self-preservation that drives them to prolong their own lives whenever possible.

Self-preservation is the most powerful instinct in existence, and thus presumed to be the strongest of all possible interests an organism can have. In comparison, the satisfaction of personal vanity in humans through breeding seems considerably less significant, more alike the modern wearing of fur coats than the slaughtering of animals for human consumption.

If, in conclusion, we consider quality of life under the aspect of maximising the animals' well-being, and presuming that animal husbandry conditions in purebred dog breeding and owning are usually of satisfactory quality, it should also be stated that dogs would have considerably more occasions for well-being during a longer lifespan than they have during a shorter one.

7.3.3 Hereditary Diseases

Hereditary diseases have been reported to occur in almost all dog breeds and also in mongrels, and their frequency and distribution varies depending on the breeds and families considered (Peyer 1997; Ackerman 1999; Ruvinsky and Sampson 2001). More and more such diseases continue to be identified, and it is entirely possible that this will also affect Irish Wolfhounds in the future. Given these facts, it is unlikely that the domestic dog population will ever be entirely free from hereditary diseases; however, few would agree that the mere occurrence of hereditary diseases in a breed of dog renders breeding the said breed unethical in itself. A certain percentage of the hereditary disease cases that occur in breeding can therefore be considered to be unfortunate, but inevitable.

Nevertheless, much of what has been said in the previous chapters is equally applicable to the case of hereditary diseases insofar as they can be taken as examples where human and animal interests are opposing. In addition to the problem of a shortened lifespan, we are also confronted with suffering due to both the diseases in themselves and, in some cases and transiently, to their veterinary treatment.

An ethical consideration that is more specific to the problem of hereditary diseases would be the fact that the influence of personal breeding choices on their rate of occurrence is usually defined more clearly than is the case with lifespan. In this context, it is possible for a stud dog to be a documented carrier of a hereditary disease, but to also produce show-winning offspring at the same time. However, this is essentially another situation in which the human interest to satisfy one's own vanity must be ranked lower than the dogs' primary interest not to suffer from a particular hereditary disease, with all the resulting ethical implications discussed in the previous chapter.

The question of hereditary diseases should also be addressed with regard to the circumstances that lead to their occurrence. Hereditary diseases, being genetic and therefore essentially stochastic in nature, can occasionally occur despite optimal selection against them having taken place. The ethical issues begin once the dogs' welfare interests are deliberately or negligently superseded by the human interest of satisfying one's emotional and/or monetary interests in selection. The inherent absurdity of this concept may best be illustrated by asking the question of how many cases of hereditary disease are worth a show champion. A special and exemplary case of this is discussed in the following chapter.

7.3.4 Portosystemic Shunt: Study of A Special Case

As mentioned in chapter 3.2.3, the problem of PSS represents a peculiar ethical dilemma that to the author's knowledge has not been reported in other hereditary diseases to-date, even though it has been published beforehand that Irish Wolfhound breeders were not realising the full potential of selection against the condition (Ubbink, van de Broeck et al. 1998).

As shown in chapter 3.2.1.3, PSS can be diagnosed at an early age through routine blood testing (Kerr and van Doorn 1999), giving breeders the possibility of testing their litters before sale, but has a high lethality rate even when properly treated (Papazoglou, Monnet et al. 2002). Given its mode of inheritance (van Steenbeek, Leegwater et al. 2009), both parents of an affected individual are identified as carriers, while healthy full siblings can be expected to carry a two-third risk of also being carriers.

Hereditary diseases of which the symptoms first appear only after the affected dog has been sold can cause concerns to both the breeder and the new owner and have – apart from the emotional distress involved for both parties – a potential for legal and financial consequences (e.g. costs of therapy, damage lawsuits). The prevention of such cases is obviously in the legitimate interest of both breeders and buyers, and a pre-sale screening test for a disease known to occur in a breed is a useful instrument to reach this goal.

However, the availability of such a screening test, possibly combined with an overestimation of treatment success rates as well as an underestimation of the suffering involved for affected dogs, can lead breeders and breeding associations to the conclusion that screening puppies before sale is a sufficient preventive measure against the problems caused by the condition, and that selection measures against the use of healthy carriers are therefore not necessary.

It is also possible to argue that affected individuals could be euthanised immediately after diagnosis, thus sparing them any medically relevant suffering. While this is technically correct, the practice becomes ethically problematic when combined with the continuous use of healthy carriers in breeding: It is accepted that breeding will result in a certain percentage of puppies "born as waste" that could have been reduced by proper selection of breeding stock. This is a practical example of the Cartesian view of animals as mentioned in chapter 7.3.1.2, in which the dogs are essentially considered expendable goods rather than living beings of an inherent ethical value.

It is obvious that a disease that kills affected dogs before breeding age must be transmitted through healthy carriers, and that the mere elimination of affected individuals will therefore not reduce its incidence in the population. However, the presence of a screening test that recognises affected puppies has the potential to encourage the use of known carriers for breeding, thus spreading the defective allele throughout the breeding population and having the potential of actually increasing the incidence of the disease in the medium to long term.

Thus, incorporating a PSS screening test into a breeders' club's code of ethics or breeding regulations cannot, in itself, be considered to be a particularly ethical act unless it is combined with the requirement to exclude the healthy carriers thus identified from breeding. The abuse of routine screening to primarily serve the breeders' and buyers' rather than the dog population's interests demonstrates another conflict of interests as specified in chapter 7.3.1.

In conclusion, the case study of PSS in Irish Wolfhounds shows the ethical importance of not merely using the available screening methods to serve human interests, but also taking their genetic consequences into consideration when selecting breeding stock.

7.4 Future Prospects in Breeding

7.4.1 General Considerations

The findings presented in this study show that Irish Wolfhounds are subject to a decrease in average lifespan as well as a number of hereditary diseases and diseases with a hereditary component, and that lifespan in the breed has decreased markedly since the 1960s. While this is likely due to a number of concurrent factors, the decrease in selection pressure for health traits is common to the majority of them (see chapter 7.1.4). Thus, it suggests itself to return towards more severe selection strategies for physical vigour in order to allow the population to get back to the level of genetic and, consequently, physical fitness that it possessed in the early 1960s through continuous purging of deleterious alleles. If a mean Irish Wolfhound lifespan of 8.92 ± 2.23 years was possible to reach in the past, it should also be possible to reach in the future.

A common argument against rigorous selection for vigour traits – rigorous selection in general – in Irish Wolfhounds is the allegation that the gene pool of the breed is too small for it to survive such measures. However, the results of the study at hand make it quite clear that, given the apparent lack of inbreeding influence on lifespan as well as the exponential increase in population size over time, the potential for severe health- and vigour-based selection was never as good in the breed as it is at present, as the number of potential breeding animals on which to base selection is higher than ever before.

Practically, and apart from measures against specific hereditary diseases, this would imply the exclusion of dogs from breeding that get affected by medical conditions that would likely have killed them in earlier times, such as e.g. severe infections. This does not imply that one should leave such dogs without proper veterinary care, but rather that such facts from potential breeding animals' medical histories should be remembered as selection criteria even after the animals have recovered. The tendency of kennels to have fewer bitches and a smaller overall number of litters is another example of breeders' and population interests being opposed in this aspect of selection (see chapter 7.3.1.2).

The present population is subject to at least two potential bottleneck events that have taken place since the times of dog 5838 due to the excessive use of two particular stud dogs – one used at least 41 times between 1972 and 1977, the other also used at least 41 times between 1993 and 2005 and one of its full brothers used at least 23 times between 1995 and 2002. These would represent the first two bottlenecks in the population history during which the breed has no longer been under considerable natural selection pressure, which may have decreased purging.

7.4.2 Hereditary Diseases

Selection decisions against hereditary diseases should be based on their frequency in the population, the severity of suffering they cause in the affected dogs, the ease of diagnosis, and the mode of inheritance. In this context, it seems reasonable to concentrate selection efforts on conditions that are widespread throughout the population, cause severe suffering and/or death, can be diagnosed easily (making screening possible) and have a high heritability, since selection against such conditions can be expected to potentially yield the highest benefit.

While there are currently no hereditary diseases in Irish Wolfhounds that can be diagnosed using a DNA test, two conditions in particular do fulfil the requirements specified above: DCM and PSS.

DCM has a high level of prevalence, undoubtedly causes suffering and death in the dog (and considerable veterinary costs for the owner), can be easily diagnosed through the published ultrasonography reference values, and has a published mode of inheritance. The disadvantage is that it cannot be diagnosed from birth onwards, but rather manifests itself in dogs that are past the age at which the first breeding usually takes place, which implies that ultrasound screening needs to be repeated throughout the breeding career of the animal and also thereafter, since symptoms of hereditary DCM can still appear at a relatively late age. The approach of using frozen semen of dead sires known to have been DCM-free throughout their lives up to old age could be a potential means of omitting this problem (see chapter 7.4.3).

PSS has a high allele frequency in the population, causes an important degree of suffering and, potentially, death in affected animals (and also considerable costs for treatment), can be diagnosed at an early age through routine screening, and its mode of inheritance renders the indirect identification of carriers possible through the screening of their direct progeny.

Where other diseases follow a defined mode of inheritance (PCD, vWD, PRA, Epilepsy), control measures based on the points mentioned in chapter three suggest themselves. As for the major diseases with hereditary components (OS, GDV and, depending on the actual prevalence, OC), the establishing of multi-parametric selection based on BLUP-estimated breeding values derived from a central health registry would be the means of choice (also see chapter 7.4.4).

However, it is also important to stress out that the prevalence levels of hereditary diseases may vary between different populations, which may lead to differences in the most appropriate selection strategy for a given population (also see chapter 6.2.7). Given the amount of genetic afflictions in the breed, it is impossible to recommend a general strategy that will be applicable to all populations. Nevertheless, the information concerning modes of inheritance and control measures mentioned in chapter 3 will hopefully give a solid base on which to develop breeding programs that are adapted to different populations' specific needs. Working to make solid health data on which to base such strategies available is of paramount importance in this context (also see chapter 7.4.4 below).

7.4.3 Lifespan

It has been shown that there are genetic contributions to canine lifespan per se (Canterberry, Greer et al. 2005), but their influence independent from hereditary disease predispositions remains unclear. The differences found between direct progeny of popular sires in this study (see chapter 6.2.5) are an indication towards such an effect, but insufficient as proof. Heredity of working lifespan has been investigated in German Shepherds and Labrador Retrievers used as guide dogs (Cole 2003), but the heritability values found were low (h^2 = 0.016 to 0.032). Since working lifespan and effective lifespan are not necessarily identical, the significance of these findings to Irish Wolfhounds remains unclear.

Some breeders are currently employing the technique of using frozen semen of dogs that are known to have lived to a certain age in the hope of increasing the lifespan of the progeny produced. This is an interesting approach, given that it removes the uncertainty associated with the use of a young stud dog regarding his medical history. However, its concrete effects on the lifespan of progeny depend on the heritability of longevity, as well as the ability to reconstruct the dogs' life medical histories in order to be able to select for vigour and to omit hereditary diseases.

Depending on the heredity of lifespan in itself, it would be possible to establish Estimation of Breeding Values (BLUP) for lifespan and vigour parameters, based not only on the longevity of a particular sire, but also on the longevity of its parents, siblings and offspring. However, the chance of success of this approach again largely depends on the heritability of lifespan itself, which remains to be assessed.

Given the currently prevailing theory of decreased lifespan in large dogs being caused by an "oxidative burst" during the rapid growth phase (see chapter 7.1.1), another approach with the potential to increase lifespan may be the selection towards a slower growth rate early in life. However, there is a chance that this may pose a conflict with the desired end height.

7.4.4 Conclusion

While it will probably be impossible to entirely eliminate every hereditary disease from the Irish Wolfhound gene pool, it seems feasible to diminish their frequency by an important degree if breeders are willing to select against them. It seems likewise possible to increase average lifespan in the breed back to the levels where it was in the 1960s if appropriate selection for vigour traits is also included in breeding strategy. There is no evidence to suggest that the breeding population is too small for rigorous selection to be possible – much to the contrary –, but individual breeders' motivation to use their particular bitches and/or stud dogs for breeding may pose a problem.

Establishing an international open pedigree-linked health database would be an invaluable means for selection to improve health and longevity in the breed, but would need coordinated international cooperation as well as openness on the breeders' part concerning health problems in their dogs. Ultimately, coordinated breeding efforts imply a decrease of personal autonomy in selection, which, given its contradiction to some breeders' personal interests, will likely result in practical problems in establishing such efforts. Nevertheless, it currently seems to be the only way through which health and lifespan could be potentially improved within the breed and thus warrants further efforts to be undertaken in this direction. As demonstrated in the study at hand, it is possible to accumulate in-depth pedigree and health information. Getting permission to publish the health-related parts, however, poses some practical difficulties.

7.5 Future Research Prospects

7.5.1 General

To the author's knowledge, this is the first study endeavouring to document the genetic structure of a breed of dog throughout its modern history. Thanks to the ever-increasing possibilities of worldwide communication through the internet, it has become possible to locate fanciers who have invested their time in creating vast pedigree databases on their respective breeds. While these databases can vary in both quality and completeness as well as their creators' willingness to cooperate in a research project, they represent a potentially invaluable resource for genetic research. This will hopefully result in similar studies in other companion animal breeds in the future.

The methods used in this study showed Pedigree Explorer® (de Jong 2002-2006) to be a useful software to convert a large existing database into a sufficient quality for genetic analysis by providing automatic detection of double entries, similar names, time-related inconsistencies etc. Given its usefulness for general pedigree data management and its compatibility with other commonly used database programs, there is no reason why it should not find further applications in future genetic research.

Nowadays, many breed clubs make use of the estimation of Breeding Values as a means of selection, combining pedigree and health data for evaluation with the BLUP method. The more accurate information is known, the better the results of such estimations – which includes pedigree information. Thus, there is a distinct potential for the application of large pedigree databases in this field.

Another field where much research remains to be undertaken is the genetics of lifespan in the domestic dog. While aging-related loci have been published (Canterberry, Greer et al. 2005), studies assessing the heritability of lifespan in the dog are still missing in the literature.

Given the current theory of an oxidative mechanism of aging during the growth phase in large dogs (see chapter 7.1.1), it would also be interesting to study the effects of treatments with antioxidant substances administered during the growth phase on life expectancy in these dogs.

7.5.2 Irish Wolfhounds

Based on the present data, a more extensive evaluation of the genetics of lifespan per se in Irish Wolfhounds would be an interesting possibility. Software packages such as The Survival Kit® have been successfully used on dog populations to assess genetic influences on working lifespan (Cole 2003), and similar work could also be carried out on overall lifespan in Irish Wolfhounds using the present data.

While the detected lack of negative inbreeding effects on lifespan and causes of death in the databases used for this study is an interesting finding, it would be equally interesting to study fertility parameters in relation to the level of inbreeding (Hedrick and Kalinowski 2000). Since our present data did neither contain records of failed matings nor consistently complete information on litter size and peripartal mortality, it was impossible to assess a possible influence of inbreeding on these parameters as described in the literature. Given that many breed clubs keep such records in their archives, it would be interesting to combine the present database with information on these fertility parameters to further analyse possible inbreeding effects in Irish Wolfhounds. This was achieved in practice using Irish Wolfhound breeding data collected by the Swedish Kennel Club from 1976 to 2007. The resulting paper (Urfer 2009) has been added to the appendix of this study

The mathematical analysis of pedigree data is an important part of genetic research, and large pedigree databases also constitute a powerful tool in searching for molecular markers for certain hereditary conditions. While it was possible to document the heredity of certain diseases in the present data, the lack of information on complete litters made it impossible to determine exact modes of inheritance. It would therefore be an interesting possibility to combine the pedigree information in the present database with health data on complete litters to study modes of inheritance.

The present database could also serve as a useful base for the establishment of index selection based on estimation of breeding values using BLUP models. Given the points specified above, it would be important to try and include information on complete litters whenever possible in future databases.

8 References

Ackerman, L. (1999). The Genetic Connection - A Guide to Health Problems in Purebred Dogs. Lakewood, Colorado, AAHA Publishing.
Adams, D. and J. Gillespie (1979). "Restoration of an incisor tooth of a Wolfhound: case report." J Small Anim Pract **20**(11): 691-5.
Aklog, L., M. P. Murphy, et al. (1994). "Right latissimus dorsi cardiomyoplasty improves left ventricular function by increasing peak systolic elastance (Emax)." Circulation **90**(5 Pt 2): II112-9.
Allgoewer, I., M. Blair, et al. (2000). "Extraocular muscle myositis and restrictive strabismus in 10 dogs." Vet Ophthalmol **3**(1): 21-26.
Anonymous (1922-2005). Irish Wolfhound Club [of the UK] Yearbooks.
Anonymous (2002). [Breeding Regulations of the IWCS]. Basel.
Anonymous. (2005 a). "[Breeding Regulations of the DWZRV]." Retrieved 17. Nov, from http://www.dwzrv.de/verband/organisation/zuchtord/zuchtordnung.htm.
Anonymous. (2005 b). "OFA Statistics and Data - Irish Wolfhound." Retrieved May 8, 2006, from http://www.offa.org/stats.html#breed.
Ashton, J. A., J. P. Farese, et al. (2005). "Investigation of the effect of pamidronate disodium on the in vitro viability of osteosarcoma cells from dogs." Am J Vet Res **66**(5): 885-91.
Ayroles, J. F., K. A. Hughes, et al. (2009). "A genomewide assessment of inbreeding depression: gene number, function, and mode of action." Conserv Biol **23**(4): 920-30.
Bech-Nielsen, S., M. E. Haskins, et al. (1978). "Frequency of osteosarcoma among first-degree relatives of St. Bernard dogs." J Natl Cancer Inst **60**(2): 349-53.
Bernardi, G. (1986). "Longevity and Morbidity in the Irish Wolfhound in the United States - 1966 to 1986." AKC Gazette **105**: 70-78.
Bernhardt, N., A. Westhoff, et al. (1996). "[Scintigraphic study for the diagnosis of portosystemic shunts in dogs]." Dtsch Tierarztl Wochenschr **103**(5): 183-6.
Bishop, L. (1986). "Ultrastructural investigations of cardiomyopathy in the dog." J Comp Pathol **96**(6): 685-98.
Bodey, A. R. and A. R. Michell (1996). "Epidemiological study of blood pressure in domestic dogs." J Small Anim Pract **37**(3): 116-25.
Bohn, F. K., D. F. Patterson, et al. (1971). "Atrial fibrillation in dogs." Br Vet J **127**(10): 485-96.
Borenstein, N., V. Chetboul, et al. (2002). "Successful cellular cardiomyoplasty in canine idiopathic dilated cardiomyopathy." Ann Thorac Surg **74**(1): 298-9; author reply 299.
Bright, J. M. and M. Dentino (2002). "Indirect arterial blood pressure measurement in nonsedated Irish Wolfhounds: reference values for the breed." J Am Anim Hosp Assoc **38**(6): 521-6.
Broome, C. J., V. P. Walsh, et al. (2004). "Congenital portosystemic shunts in dogs and cats." N Z Vet J **52**(4): 154-62.
Broschk, C. C. (2004). Analyse der Populationsstruktur und populationsgenetische Untersuchung zur Vererbung der dilatativen Kardiomyopathie beim Irischen Wolfshund. DVM Thesis, TIHO Hannover.
Brownlie, S. and H. Nott (1991). "An investigation of size in Irish Wolfhounds with supraventricular cardiac arrhythmias." Vet Rec **129**(22): 493.
Brownlie, S. E. (1991). "An electrocardiographic survey of cardiac rhythm in Irish Wolfhounds." Vet Rec **129**(21): 470-1.

Brownlie, S. E. and M. A. Cobb (1999). "Observations on the development of congestive heart failure in Irish Wolfhounds with dilated cardiomyopathy." J Small Anim Pract **40**(8): 371-7.

Brunnberg, L., M. Burger, et al. (2005). [Surgery of Hereditary Orthopaedic Diseases]. Proceedings of the 20th VK Annual Meeting, Salzburg, pp. 107-115.

Burrows, C. F. and L. A. Ignaszweski (1990). "Canine gastric dilatation-volvulus." J Small Anim Pract **31**: 495-501.

Canterberry, S. C., K. A. Greer, et al. (2005). "Aging-associated loci in Canis familiaris." Growth Dev Aging **69**(2): 101-13.

Casal, M. L. (2004). "Wolfhound Rhinitis/Primary Ciliary Dyskinesia." Retrieved March 15, 2006, from http://www.irishwolfhoundstudy.com/pcd/casal.htm.

Casal, M. L. and P. S. Henthorn. (2008). "PCD & Epilepsy Update: May, 2008." Retrieved August 9, 2009, from http://www.irishwolfhoundstudy.com/pcd/snip.htm.

Casal, M. L., R. M. Munuve, et al. (2006). "Epilepsy in Irish Wolfhounds." J Vet Intern Med **20**(1): 131-5.

Casal, M. L., P. Werner, et al. (2009). "Idiopathic Epilepsy in the Irish Wolfhound: Update May 4, 2009." Retrieved August 9th, 2009, from http://www.irishwolfhoundstudy.com/seizures/idio.htm.

Charlesworth, D. and B. Charlesworth (1987). "Inbreeding Depression and its Evolutionary Consequences." Annu Rev Ecol Syst **18**: 237-68.

Chun, R., L. D. Garrett, et al. (2005). "Toxicity and Efficacy of Cisplatin and Doxorubicin Combination Chemotherapy for the Treatment of Canine Osteosarcoma." J Am Anim Hosp Assoc **41**(6): 382-387.

Chun, R. and W. B. Morrison (2004). Osteosarcoma. in: The 5-Minute Veterinary Consult: Canine and Feline, 3rd ed. pp. 950-1. L. P. Tilley and F. W. K. Smith, Lippincott Williams & Williams.

Clark, P. and B. W. Parry (1995). "Survey of Irish Wolfhounds in Australia for von Willebrand's disease." Aust Vet J **72**(10): 393.

Clark, P. and B. W. Parry (1997). "Some haematological values of Irish Wolfhounds in Australia." Aust Vet J **75**(7): 523-4.

Clercx, C., I. Reichler, et al. (2003). "Rhinitis/Bronchopneumonia syndrome in Irish Wolfhounds." J Vet Intern Med **17**(6): 843-9.

Cobb, M. A., S. Brownlie, et al. (1996). Evidence for genetic involvement in dilated cardiomyopathy in the Irish Wolfhound. Brit Sm Anim Vet Assoc Congress, Birmingham, April:215.

Cole, J. B. (2003). Population Structure and Genetics of Longevity in a Colony of Dog Guides. Agricultural and Mechanical College. Biton Rouge, Louisiana State University.

Comfort, A. (1956). "Longevity and Mortality of Irish Wolfhounds." Proc Zoolog Soc London **CXXVII**(Sept. 1956, Part 1): 27-34.

Comfort, A. (1960). "Longevity and Mortality in Dogs of Four Breeds." J Gerontol **15 A**: 126-9.

Connery, N. A., H. McAllister, et al. (2002). "Cellophane banding of congenital intrahepatic portosystemic shunts in two Irish Wolfhounds." J Small Anim Pract **43**(8): 345-9.

Cooley, D. M., B. C. Beranek, et al. (2002). "Endogenous gonadal hormone exposure and bone sarcoma risk." Cancer Epidemiol Biomarkers Prev **11**(11): 1434-40.

Crnokrak, P. and S. C. Barrett (2002). "Perspective: purging the genetic load: a review of the experimental evidence." Evolution Int J Org Evolution **56**(12): 2347-58.

Crookshanks, J. L., S. M. Taylor, et al. (2007). "Treatment of canine pediatric Neospora caninum myositis following immunohistochemical identification of tachyzoites in muscle biopsies." Can Vet J **48**(5): 506-8.

Dahlbom, M., M. Andersson, et al. (1995). "Poor semen quality in Irish Wolfhounds: a clinical, hormonal and spermatological study." J Small Anim Pract **36**(12): 547-52.

Dahlbom, M., M. Andersson, et al. (1997). "Fertility parameters in male Irish Wolfhounds: a two-year follow-up study." J Small Anim Pract **38**(12): 547-50.

de Jong, R. (2002-2006). Pedigree Explorer - program for the management of pedigree data; http://www.breedmate.com.

Deeb, B. and N. Wolf (1994). "Studying longevity and morbidity in giant and small breeds of dogs." Vet Med **89**(Aug 1994 Sup Geriatric Med): 702-13.

DeQuoy, A. W. (1971). The Irish Wolfhound in Irish literature and law. McLean, Va.,.

DeQuoy, A. W. (1973). The Irish Wolfhound guide. [Dublin,, Printed by Cahill].

DeQuoy, A. W. (1991). Modern wolf and Irish Wolfhound skeletons. [McLean, Va.?], A. DeQuoy.

DeQuoy, A. W., G. d. Q. Castillo, et al. (1993). Irish Wolfhound saga : a trilogy. [McLean, VA?], A. de Q.

Distl, O., A. C. Vollmar, et al. (2007). "Complex segregation analysis of dilated cardiomyopathy (DCM) in Irish wolfhounds." Heredity **99**(4): 460-5.

Donnelly, J. P. (1976). Wolfhound Longevity. in: Raising, Showing and Breeding the Irish Wolfhound. E. C. Murphy. Dublin, Richview Press, Ltd.: pp. 302-3.

Dorn, C. R. (2002). Canine breed-specific risks of frequently diagnosed diseases at veterinary teaching hospitals, AKC Canine Health Foundation.

Douglas, S. W. and D. F. Kelly (1966). "Calcinosis circumscripta of the tongue." J Small Anim Pract **7**(6): 441-3.

Doyle, A. K. (2002). A Discussion of the Irish Wolfhound. Cavan, Privately published.

Dyce, J. and J. E. F. Houlton (1993). "Fibrocartilaginous Embolism in the Dog." J Small Anim Pract **34**: 332-6.

Edwards, D. F. and L. R. Johnson (2004). Primary Ciliary Dyskinesia. in: The 5-Minute Veterinary Consult: Canine and Feline, 3rd ed. pp. 1061-2. L. P. Tilley and F. W. K. Smith, Lippincott Williams & Williams.

Egenvall, A., B. N. Bonnett, et al. (2006). "Heart disease as a cause of death in insured Swedish dogs younger than 10 years of age." J Vet Intern Med **20**(4): 894-903.

Egenvall, A., B. N. Bonnett, et al. (2005). "Mortality in over 350,000 insured Swedish dogs from 1995-2000: II. Breed-specific age and survival patterns and relative risk for causes of death." Acta Vet Scand **46**(3): 121-36.

Egenvall, A., A. Nodtvedt, et al. (2007). "Bone tumors in a population of 400 000 insured Swedish dogs up to 10 y of age: incidence and survival." Can J Vet Res **71**(4): 292-9.

Ettinger, S. J., A. M. Benitz, et al. (1998). "Effects of enalapril maleate on survival of dogs with naturally acquired heart failure. The Long-Term Investigation of Veterinary Enalapril (LIVE) Study Group." J Am Vet Med Assoc **213**(11): 1573-7.

Ettinger, S. J. and E. C. Feldman (1995). Textbok of Veterinary Internal Medicine, 4th Edition. Philadelphia, W.B. Saunders Company, pp. 644-9 and 2050-1.

Fan, T. M., L. P. de Lorimier, et al. (2005). "Evaluation of intravenous pamidronate administration in 33 cancer-bearing dogs with primary or secondary bone involvement." J Vet Intern Med **19**(1): 74-80.

Farese, J. P., J. Ashton, et al. (2004). "The effect of the bisphosphonate alendronate on viability of canine osteosarcoma cells in vitro." In Vitro Cell Dev Biol Anim **40**(3-4): 113-7.

Ferracini, R., P. Angelini, et al. (2000). "MET oncogene aberrant expression in canine osteosarcoma." J Orthop Res **18**(2): 253-6.

Fossum, T. W. and C. S. Hedlund (2002). Portosystemic Shunts. in: Small animal surgery. St. Louis, Mosby: p. 820 ff.

Fowler, K. and M. C. Whitlock (1999). "The variance in inbreeding depression and the recovery of fitness in bottlenecked populations." Proc Biol Sci **266**(1433): 2061-6.

Fox, P. R., D. Sisson, et al. (1999). Textbook of canine and feline cardiology : principles and clinical practice. Philadelphia, Pa., Saunders.

Fuentes, V. L., B. Corcoran, et al. (2002). "A double-blind, randomized, placebo-controlled study of pimobendan in dogs with dilated cardiomyopathy." J Vet Intern Med **16**(3): 255-61.

Galis, F., I. Van Der Sluijs, et al. (2006). "Do large dogs die young?" J Exp Zoolog B Mol Dev Evol.

Gardner, P. (1931). The Irish Wolfhound; a short historical sketch. Dundalk,, The Dundalgan press.

Gelatt, K. N. and E. O. Mackay (2005). "Prevalence of primary breed-related cataracts in the dog in North America." Vet Ophthalmol **8**(2): 101-11.

Gerritzen-Bruning, M. J., T. S. van den Ingh, et al. (2006). "Diagnostic value of fasting plasma ammonia and bile acid concentrations in the identification of portosystemic shunting in dogs." J Vet Intern Med **20**(1): 13-9.

Glickman, L. T., N. W. Glickman, et al. (2000 b). "Non-dietary risk factors for gastric dilatation-volvulus in large and giant breed dogs." J Am Vet Med Assoc **217**(10): 1492-9.

Glickman, L. T., N. W. Glickman, et al. (2000 a). "Incidence of and breed-related risk factors for gastric dilatation-volvulus in dogs." J Am Vet Med Assoc **216**(1): 40-5.

Gould, D. J., S. M. Petersen-Jones, et al. (1997). "Cloning of canine rom-1 and its investigation as a candidate gene for generalized progressive retinal atrophies in dogs." Anim Genet **28**(6): 391-6.

Gover, L. (1998). The Irish Wolfhound. London, Kingdom Books.

Graham, G. A. (1885). The Irish Wolfhound. Dursley [Gloucestershire], Whitmore & Son.

Graham, G. A. (1906/1959). Irish Wolfhound Pedigrees 1859-1906. River Valley, Irish Wolfhound Club of Ireland.

Greer, K. A., S. C. Canterberry, et al. (2006). "Statistical analysis regarding the effects of height and weight on life span of the domestic dog." Res Vet Sci.

Harpster, N. K. (1994). Cardiac Arrhythmias in the Irish Wolfhound: Preliminary Study. Proceedings of the 12th ACVIM Forum, San Francisco, CA, pp. 319-324.

Hedrick, P. W. and S. T. Kalinowski (2000). "Inbreeding Depression in Conservation Biology." Annu Rev Ecol Syst **31**: 139-62.

Heffels, D. (1989). Irish Wolfhound. Schnelldorf, Selisch Verlag.

Herden, C., A. Beineke, et al. (2003). "Unusual manifestation of hepatic encephalopathy in two Irish Wolfhound siblings." Vet Rec **153**(22): 682-6.

Heuch, I. and F. H. Li (1972). "PEDIG--a computer program for calculation of genotype probabilities using phenotype information." Clin Genet 3(6): 501-4.

Hogan, E. (1897). The Irish Wolfdog. Dublin, Sealy, Bryers & Walker ; M.H. Gill & Son.

Hudson, D. E. S. (1981). The Brabyns Handbook on Irish Wolfhounds. Woking, Surrey, Optichrome, Ltd.

Hunt, G. B. (2004). "Effect of breed on anatomy of portosystemic shunts resulting from congenital diseases in dogs and cats: a review of 242 cases." Aust Vet J 82(12): 746-9.

Johnson, A. S., C. G. Couto, et al. (1998). "Mutation of the p53 tumor suppressor gene in spontaneously occurring osteosarcomas of the dog." Carcinogenesis 19(1): 213-7.

Junker, K., T. S. van den Ingh, et al. (2000). "Fibrocartilaginous embolism of the spinal cord (FCE) in juvenile Irish Wolfhounds." Vet Q 22(3): 154-6.

Kalbfleisch, J. D. and R. L. Prentice (1980). The Statistical Analysis of FailureTime Data, Wiley Series in Probability and Mathematical Statistics.

Kalinowski, S. T., P. W. Hedrick, et al. (2000). "Inbreeding Depression in the Speke's Gazelle Captive Breeding Program." Conservation Biology 14(5): 1375-1384.

Kane, A. (2001). Irish Wolfhound. Dorking, Surrey, Interpet Publishing.

Kealy, R. D., D. F. Lawler, et al. (2002). "Effects of diet restriction on life span and age-related changes in dogs." J Am Vet Med Assoc 220(9): 1315-20.

Kerr, M. G. (1996). "Hyperammonaemia in Irish Wolfhounds." Vet Rec 138(7): 167-8.

Kerr, M. G. and T. van Doorn (1999). "Mass screening of Irish Wolfhound puppies for portosystemic shunts by the dynamic bile acid test." Vet Rec 144(25): 693-6.

Kirkpatrick, M. and P. Jarne (2000). "The Effects of a Bottleneck on Inbreeding Depression and the Genetic Load." Am Nat 155(2): 154-167.

Koch, J., H. D. Pedersen, et al. (1996). "M-mode echocardiographic diagnosis of dilated cardiomyopathy in giant breed dogs." Zentralbl Veterinarmed A 43(5): 297-304.

Kociba, G. J. and S. A. Kruth (2004). Von Willebrand Disease. in: The 5-Minute Veterinary Consult: Canine and Feline, 3rd ed. pp. 1362-3. L. P. Tilley and F. W. K. Smith, Lippincott Williams & Williams.

Kraft, W. (2000). [Diagnostic Measures for Liver Disease]. in: [Small Animal Diseases]. Stuttgart, Verlag Eugen Ulmer. 1: p. 575.

Kramer, M. T., K. S. Latimer, et al. (2003). "Canine Osteosarcoma." Retrieved 3.Jan, 2006, from http://www.msu.edu/~silvar/osteosarcoma.htm.

Krohne, S. (2001). "Inherited Cataracts in Dogs." Canine Eye Registry Foundation Newsletter(August).

Lacy, R. C., G. Alaks, et al. (1996). "Hierarchical Analysis of Inbreeding Depression in Peromyscus Polionotus." Evolution Int J Org Evolution 50(6): 2187-2200.

Lacy, R. C. and J. D. Ballou (1998). "Effectiveness of Selection in Reducing the Genetic Load in Populations of Peromyscus Polionotus During Generations of Inbreeding." Evolution Int J Org Evolution 52(3): 900-909.

Lawler, D. F., R. H. Evans, et al. (2005). "Influence of lifetime food restriction on causes, time, and predictors of death in dogs." J Am Vet Med Assoc 226(2): 225-31.

Leisewitz, A. L., J. A. Spencer, et al. (1997). "Suspected primary immunodeficiency syndrome in three related Irish Wolfhounds." J Small Anim Pract 38(5): 209-12.

Leveille, R., S. E. Johnson, et al. (2003). "Transvenous coil embolization of portosystemic shunt in dogs." Vet Radiol Ultrasound 44(1): 32-6.

Levine, R. A., T. Forest, et al. (2002). "Tumor suppressor PTEN is mutated in canine osteosarcoma cell lines and tumors." Vet Pathol **39**(3): 372-8.

Li, Y., B. Deeb, et al. (1996). "Cellular proliferative capacity and life span in small and large dogs." J Gerontol A Biol Sci Med Sci **51**(6): B403-8.

Maison, F. P. N. (1990). Contribution ι l'tude de l'Irish Wolfhound. Facult Vtrinaire. Toulouse, Universit Paul Sabatier: 123.

Mathew, L. and S. D. Katz (1998). "Calcium sensitising agents in heart failure." Drugs Aging **12**(3): 191-204.

McBryde, M. (1998). Magnificient Irish Wolfhound, the. Dorking, Ringpress Books.

Mendoza, S., T. Konishi, et al. (1998). "Status of the p53, Rb and MDM2 genes in canine osteosarcoma." Anticancer Res **18**(6A): 4449-53.

Meyer, B., H. Murua Escobar, et al. (2004). "Expression pattern of the HMGB1 gene in sarcomas of the dog." Anticancer Res **24**(2B): 707-10.

Meyer, H. P., J. Rothuizen, et al. (1996). "Transient metabolic hyperammonaemia in young Irish Wolfhounds." Vet Rec **138**(5): 105-7.

Meyer, H. P., J. Rothuizen, et al. (1995). "Increasing incidence of hereditary intrahepatic portosystemic shunts in Irish Wolfhounds in The Netherlands (1984 to 1992)." Vet Rec **136**(1): 13-6.

Michell, A. R. (1999). "Longevity of British breeds of dog and its relationships with sex, size, cardiovascular variables and disease." Vet Rec **145**(22): 625-9.

Miller, C. H., J. B. Graham, et al. (1979 a). "Genetics of classic von Willebrand's disease. I. Phenotypic variation within families." Blood **54**(1): 117-36.

Miller, C. H., J. B. Graham, et al. (1979 b). "Genetics of classic von Willebrand's disease. II. Optimal assignment of the heterozygous genotype (diagnosis) by discriminant analysis." Blood **54**(1): 137-45.

Miller, C. O. (1988). Gazehounds: The Search for Truth. Wheat Ridge, Colorado, Hoflin Publishing, Ltd.

Monnet, E. and E. C. Orton (1994). "Dynamic cardiomyoplasty for dilated cardiomyopathy in dogs." Semin Vet Med Surg (Small Anim) **9**(4): 240-6.

Montoya, J. A., P. J. Morris, et al. (2006). "Hypertension: a risk factor associated with weight status in dogs." J Nutr **136**(7 Suppl): 2011S-2013S.

Murphy, E. C. (1991). The Irish Wolfhound: A Collection of Photographs and Pedigrees. Lucan, MarTone Press Ltd.

Murphy, E. C. (1996). "Irish Wolfhound Longevity Report." Retrieved Sept. 26, from http://www.eiwc.org/pdf/Longevity_Report.pdf.

Necas, A., M. Dvorak, et al. (1999). "Incidence of Osteochondrosis in Dogs and its Late Diagnosis." Acta Vet Brno **68**: 131-139.

Niles, J. D., J. M. Williams, et al. (2001). "Resolution of dysphagia following cricopharyngeal myectomy in six young dogs." Journal of Small Animal Practice **42**(1): 32-5.

Oh, J. H., V. Badhwar, et al. (1998). "The effects of prosthetic cardiac binding and adynamic cardiomyoplasty in a model of dilated cardiomyopathy." J Thorac Cardiovasc Surg **116**(1): 148-53.

Orton, E. C., E. Monnet, et al. (1994). "Dynamic cardiomyoplasty for treatment of idiopathic dilatative cardiomyopathy in a dog." J Am Vet Med Assoc **205**(10): 1415-9.

Osswald, S., T. G. Trouton, et al. (1998). "Transvenous single lead atrial defibrillation: efficacy and risk of ventricular fibrillation in an ischemic canine model." Pacing Clin Electrophysiol **21**(3): 580-9.

Owen, L. N. (1967). "Calcinosis circumscripta (calcium gout) in related Irish Wolfhounds." J Small Anim Pract **8**(5): 291-2.

Papazoglou, L. G., E. Monnet, et al. (2002). "Survival and prognostic indicators for dogs with intrahepatic portosystemic shunts: 32 cases (1990-2000)." Vet Surg **31**(6): 561-70.

Parent, J. M. (2004). Epilepsy, Idiopathic, Genetic, Primary. in: The 5-Minute Veterinary Consult: Canine and Feline, 3rd ed. pp. 414-5. L. P. Tilley and F. W. K. Smith, Lippincott Williams & Williams.

Patronek, G. J., D. J. Waters, et al. (1997). "Comparative longevity of pet dogs and humans: implications for gerontology research." J Gerontol A Biol Sci Med Sci **52**(3): B171-8.

Peeters, D., C. Clercx, et al. (2000). "Juvenile nephropathy in a boxer, a rottweiler, a collie and an Irish wolfhound." Aust Vet J **78**(3): 162-5.

Peyer, N. (1997). [Assessing breeding-related defects in purebred dogs for their relevance in animal protection] (Die Beurteilung zuchtbedingter Defekte bei Rassehunden in tierschützerischer Hinsicht).DVM Thesis. Veterinary Faculty, University of Bern: p. 154.

Philipp, U., C. Broschk, et al. (2007). "Evaluation of tafazzin as candidate for dilated cardiomyopathy in Irish wolfhounds." J Hered **98**(5): 506-9.

Philipp, U., A. Vollmar, et al. (2008 a). "Evaluation of the titin-cap gene (TCAP) as candidate for dilated cardiomyopathy in Irish wolfhounds." Anim Biotechnol **19**(4): 231-6.

Philipp, U., A. Vollmar, et al. (2008 b). "Evaluation of six candidate genes for dilated cardiomyopathy in Irish wolfhounds." Anim Genet **39**(1): 88-9.

Priester, W. A. and F. W. McKay (1980). "The occurrence of tumors in domestic animals." Natl Cancer Inst Monograph **54**: 169.

Prokopenko, S. e. a. (1998). "Irish Wolfhound-H Longevity Survey." Retrieved 22. 09. 2005, from http://www.netrover.com/~wolfie1/iwh/longsurv.htm.

Rothuizen, J. (2002). Molecular Genetics - Diseases of the Liver. Proceedings of the 27th WSAVA Congress, Granada, http://www.vin.com/proceedings/Proceedings.plx?CID=WSAVA2002&PID=2623&Category=419.

Ru, G., B. Terracini, et al. (1998). "Host related risk factors for canine osteosarcoma." Vet J **156**(1): 31-9.

Ruttemann, G. R. (2005). [Oncology and Genetical Predispositions] - The incidence of Tumors in Dogs and Cats and the Breed-Related Predispositions to Tumor Development. Proceedings, 20. VK-Jahrestagung, pp. 75-80, Salzburg.

Ruvinsky, A. and J. Sampson (2001). The Genetics of the Dog. Wallingford, Oxon, UK ; New York, CABI Pub.

Schawalder, P. (1997). [Dysplasias and Growth Problems]. Kleintierkrankheiten. U. f. r. Wissenschaft. Stuttgart, Eugen Ulmer & Co. **3 (Chirurgie des Bewegungsapparats)**.

Schwarz, P. D. and P. K. Shires (2004 a). Osteochondrosis. in: The 5-Minute Veterinary Consult: Canine and Feline, 3rd ed. pp. 946-7. L. P. Tilley and F. W. K. Smith, Lippincott Williams & Williams.

Schwarz, P. D. and P. K. Shires (2004 b). Elbow Dysplasia. in: The 5-Minute Veterinary Consult: Canine and Feline, 3rd ed. pp. 394-5. L. P. Tilley and F. W. K. Smith, Lippincott Williams & Williams.

Sisson, A. and J. M. Parent (2004). Fibrocartilaginous Embolic Myelopathy. in: The 5-Minute Veterinary Consult: Canine and Feline, 3rd ed. pp. 478-9. L. P. Tilley and F. W. K. Smith, Lippincott Williams & Williams.

Skancke, E. (1994). "Portosystemic shunt – persistent ductus venosus – in the Irish Wolfhound." Retrieved 28.10., 2005, from http://www.eiwc.org/pdf/Portosystemic_Shunt_in_the_IW.pdf.

Smith, P. J. and P. E. Miller (2004). Retinal Degeneration. in: The 5-Minute Veterinary Consult: Canine and Feline, 3rd ed. pp. 1136-7. L. P. Tilley and F. W. K. Smith, Lippincott Williams & Williams.

Snead, E. C. (2007). "Large granular intestinal lymphosarcoma and leukemia in a dog." Can Vet J **48**(8): 848-51.

Somerfield, F. (1998). Mission Accomplished - The Life and Times of Florence Nagle, Dogworld Publishers.

Sommerfeld-Stur, I. (2005). [Special Structure and Dynamics of Dog Populations]. Proceedings, 20. VK-Jahrestagung, Salzburg, pp. 155-160.

Starbuck, A. J. and E. S. Howell (1969). The Complete Irish Wolfhound. New York, Howell Book House.

Stokol, T., B. W. Parry, et al. (1995). "von Willebrand's disease in Dobermann dogs in Australia." Aust Vet J **72**(7): 257-62.

Suter, P. and H. G. Niemand (2001 a). [Portosystemic Shunts]. in: Praktikum der Hundeklinik. Stuttgart, Parey: p. 820 ff.

Suter, P. and H. G. Niemand (2001 b). [Osteogenic Sarcoma]. in: Praktikum der Hundeklinik. Stuttgart, Parey: p. 1218 ff.

Suter, P. and H. G. Niemand (2001 c). [Gastric Dilation Volvulus]. in: Praktikum der Hundeklinik. Stuttgart, Parey: p. 742 ff.

Symmachus, Q. A. (393). Letter to Flavianus Symmachus. in: Epistolarum ad Diversos.

Templeton, A. R. and B. Read (1984). "Factors Eliminating Inbreeding Depression in a Captive Herd of Speke's Gazelle (Gazella spekei)." Zoo Biology **3**: 177-199.

Thomas, W. B. (1994). "Managing Epileptic Dogs." The Compendium - Continuing Education, Louisiana State University School for Veterinary Medicine - Small Animals(December): 1573-1589.

Thomasson, L. J. (1999). Irish Wolfhound Odyssey : 'In Search of Graham's Hound'. [S.l.], L.J. Thomasson.

Thornhill, N. W. (1993). The Natural History of Inbreeding and Outbreeding: Theoretical and Empirical Perspectives. Chicago and London, The University of Chicago Press.

Thornton, E. S. (2005). "Progressive Retinal Atrophy (PRA)." Retrieved August 9, 2009, from http://web.archive.org/web/20060104180238/http://www.theirishwolfhound.org/health/health_zoom.asp?theid=20.

Tidholm, A. and L. Jonsson (2005). "Histologic characterization of canine dilated cardiomyopathy." Vet Pathol **42**(1): 1-8.

Tomlin, J. L., C. Sturgeon, et al. (2000). "Use of the bisphosphonate drug alendronate for palliative management of osteosarcoma in two dogs." Vet Rec **147**(5): 129-32.

Trangerud, C., J. Grondalen, et al. (2007). "A longitudinal study on growth and growth variables in dogs of four large breeds raised in domestic environments." J Anim Sci **85**(1): 76-83.

Ubbink, G. J., J. van de Broek, et al. (1998 a). "Cluster analysis of the genetic heterogeneity and disease distributions in purebred dog populations." Vet Rec **142**(9): 209-13.

Ubbink, G. J., J. van de Broek, et al. (1998 b). "Prediction of inherited portosystemic shunts in Irish Wolfhounds on the basis of pedigree analysis." American Journal of Veterinary Research **59**(12): 1553-6.

Urfer, S. and A. Steiger (2006). "Epilepsy in Irish Wolfhounds." J Vet Intern Med **20**(5): 1049; author reply 1049-51.

Urfer, S. R. (2008). "Right censored data ('cohort bias') in veterinary life span studies." Vet Rec **163**(15): 457-8.

Urfer, S. R. (2009). "Inbreeding and fertility in Irish Wolfhounds in Sweden: 1976 to 2007." Acta Vet Scand **51**: 21.

van Hagen, M. A., L. L. Janss, et al. (2004). "The use of a genetic-counselling program by Dutch breeders for four hereditary health problems in boxer dogs." Prev Vet Med **63**(1-2): 39-50.

van Leeuwen, I. S., C. J. Cornelisse, et al. (1997). "P53 gene mutations in osteosarcomas in the dog." Cancer Lett **111**(1-2): 173-8.

van Meel, J. C., A. B. Mauz, et al. (1989). "Pimobendan increases survival of cardiomyopathic hamsters." J Cardiovasc Pharmacol **13**(3): 508-9.

van Steenbeek, F. G., P. A. Leegwater, et al. (2009). "Evidence of inheritance of intrahepatic portosystemic shunts in Irish Wolfhounds." J Vet Intern Med **23**(4): 950-2.

Vaughan-Scott, T., J. Goldin, et al. (1999). "Spinal nephroblastoma in an Irish Wolfhound." J S Afr Vet Assoc **70**(1): 25-8.

Vincent, I. C. and A. R. Michell (1996). "Relationship between blood pressure and stress-prone temperament in dogs." Physiol Behav **60**(1): 135-8.

Visscher, P. M., D. Smith, et al. (2001). "A viable herd of genetically uniform cattle." Nature **409**(6818): 303.

Vollmar, A. (1996). "Kardiologische Untersuchungen beim Irischen Wolfshund unter besonderer Berücksichtigung des Vorhofflimmerns und der Echokardiographie." Kleintierpraxis(41): 393-408.

Vollmar, A. (1998). "Cardiomyopathy in the Irish Wolfhound. A clinical study of 393 dogs by electro- and echocardiography and radiology." Vet Q **20 Suppl 1**: pp.104-5.

Vollmar, A. and P. R. Fox (2001). "Clinical, echocardiographic, and ECG findings in 232 sequentially examined Irish Wolfhounds." J Vet Int Med **15**(3): 279.

Vollmar, A., P. R. Fox, et al. (2004). "Heart screening results of more than 1000 Irish Wolfhounds: Prevalence of DCM, survival characteristics, whole blood taurine & DCM inheritance. ." Retrieved Nov. 16, 2005, from http://www.eiwc.org/pdf/Heart_Problems_DCM.pdf.

Vollmar, A. C. (1999 a). "Echocardiographic measurements in the Irish wolfhound: reference values for the breed." J Am Anim Hosp Assoc **35**(4): 271-7.

Vollmar, A. C. (1999 b). "Use of echocardiography in the diagnosis of dilated cardiomyopathy in Irish wolfhounds." J Am Anim Hosp Assoc **35**(4): 279-83.

Vollmar, A. C. (2000). "The prevalence of cardiomyopathy in the Irish Wolfhound: a clinical study of 500 dogs." J Am Anim Hosp Assoc **36**(2): 125-32.

Walker, H. (1896). Der Irish Wolfhound. Schweizerisches Hundestammbuch. Bern, Schweizerische Kynologische Gesellschaft. **VI:** 64-103.

Waschak, M. J. and A. E. Jergens (2004). Gastric Dilation and Volvulus Syndrome. in: The 5-Minute Veterinary Consult: Canine and Feline, 3rd ed. pp. 492-3. L. P. Tilley and F. W. K. Smith, Lippincott Williams & Williams.

Watson, P. J. and M. E. Herrtage (1998). "Medical management of congenital portosystemic shunts in 27 dogs--a retrospective study." J Small Anim Pract **39**(2): 62-8.

Weiss, D. J. and M. Henson (2007). "Pure white cell aplasia in a dog." <u>Vet Clin Pathol</u> **36**(4): 373-5.
Weisse, C., J. I. Mondschein, et al. (2005). "Use of a percutaneous atrial septal occluder device for complete acute occlusion of an intrahepatic portosystemic shunt in a dog." <u>J Am Vet Med Assoc</u> **227**(2): 249-52, 236.
White, R. N., C. A. Burton, et al. (1998). "Surgical treatment of intrahepatic portosystemic shunts in 45 dogs." <u>Vet Rec</u> **142**(14): 358-65.
Wilkinson, G. T. (1969). "Some observations on the Irish Wolfhound Rhinitis Syndrome." <u>J Small Anim Pract</u> **10**(1): 5-8.
Williams, D. L., M. F. Heath, et al. (2004). "Prevalence of canine cataract: preliminary results of a cross-sectional study." <u>Vet Ophthalmol</u> **7**(1): 29-35.
Wolfer, J. P. (1995). <u>Acquired Strabismus in Irish Wolfhounds</u>. Proceedings of the Annual ACVO Meeting, p. 58.
Zandvliet, M. M. and J. Rothuizen (2007). "Transient hyperammonemia due to urea cycle enzyme deficiency in Irish wolfhounds." <u>J Vet Intern Med</u> **21**(2): 215-8.

9 Appendix

ID	DR	DA	DR10	DA10	GR	GA	GR10	GA10	OR	OA	OR10	OA10	PR	PA	PR10	PA10
5838	1	1	1	1	1	1	2	1	1	1	1	1	1	1	1	-
4732	2	2	2	-	2	2	1	-	2	2	2	-	2	2	-	-
4703	3	3	3	-	3	3	5	-	3	3	3	-	3	3	-	-
4605	4	4	4	-	4	4	4	-	4	5	4	-	5	5	-	-
5538	5	5	5	9	5	5	6	7	5	4	5	9	4	4	9	-
5184	6	6	6	-	6	6	7	-	6	6	6	-	6	6	-	-
5252	7	7	7	-	7	7	9	-	7	7	7	-	7	7	-	-
4681	8	8	8	-	8	8	8	-	8	8	8	-	8	8	-	-
4475	9	9	9	-	10	9	12	-	10	10	9	-	9	9	-	-
4820	10	10	10	-	12	10	-	-	12	12	12	-	10	10	-	-
6476	11	-	11	-	11	-	10	10	11	11	10	7	11	-	10	-
3132	12	11	-	-	-	11	-	-	-	-	-	-	13	-	-	-
5385	13	12	13	-	13	12	-	-	14	14	14	-	14	11	-	-
5045	14	13	14	-	14	13	19	-	15	15	15	-	15	12	-	-
4794	15	14	15	-	15	14	-	-	16	16	16	-	17	13	-	-
5273	16	15	16	-	17	16	-	-	17	17	17	-	16	15	-	-
5996	17	-	-	-	16	-	-	-	-	-	-	-	-	-	-	-
6378	18	-	18	-	18	17	-	-	-	18	20	-	-	18	-	-
4552	19	18	-	-	19	19	-	-	-	20	-	-	20	-	-	-
5548	20	19	19	-	-	-	-	-	-	-	-	-	18	19	-	-
6555	-	-	-	-	-	-	19	-	-	-	-	-	-	-	-	-
5046	-	-	-	-	-	-	-	-	-	-	-	-	-	13	-	-
6660	-	-	-	11	-	-	-	-	-	-	-	-	-	-	-	-
6661	-	-	-	12	-	-	-	14	-	-	-	18	-	-	-	-
7051	-	-	-	-	-	-	20	16	-	-	-	-	-	-	-	-
6744	-	-	-	15	-	-	-	-	-	-	-	16	-	-	-	-
7052	-	-	-	-	-	-	17	9	-	-	-	15	-	-	-	-
7617	-	-	-	-	-	-	-	-	-	-	-	-	-	-	11	-
6747	-	-	-	-	-	-	-	18	-	-	-	-	-	-	-	-
6750	-	-	-	-	-	-	-	13	-	-	-	-	-	-	-	-
6755	-	-	-	20	-	-	-	-	-	-	-	-	-	-	-	-
5117	-	-	20	-	-	-	-	-	-	-	-	-	-	-	-	-
6562	-	-	-	-	20	-	-	-	20	-	-	-	-	-	-	-
7068	-	-	-	-	-	-	-	-	-	-	-	19	-	-	-	-
7239	-	-	-	-	-	-	18	-	-	-	-	-	-	-	-	-
5625	-	-	-	-	-	-	-	-	-	-	-	17	-	-	-	-
6177	-	-	-	-	-	-	17	-	-	-	-	-	-	-	-	-
8251	-	-	-	6	-	-	-	6	-	-	-	10	-	-	6	-
9103	-	-	-	-	-	-	-	-	-	-	-	-	-	-	-	15
6180	-	-	-	16	-	-	-	-	-	-	-	-	-	-	-	-
6069	-	-	-	-	-	-	-	-	18	-	-	19	-	-	-	-
7677	-	-	-	-	-	-	-	-	-	-	-	-	-	-	18	-
7080	-	-	-	-	-	-	-	-	-	-	-	-	-	-	-	8
5283	-	17	-	-	-	18	-	-	-	-	-	-	-	-	-	-
6684	-	-	-	-	-	-	-	-	-	-	-	-	-	-	16	-
7086	-	-	-	-	-	-	-	-	-	-	-	-	-	-	-	9
5541	-	16	17	-	-	15	-	-	19	19	18	-	-	14	-	-
7978	-	-	-	5	-	-	-	-	-	-	-	-	-	-	-	7
10362	-	-	-	-	-	-	-	-	-	-	-	-	-	-	-	5
12386	-	-	-	-	-	-	-	-	-	-	-	-	-	-	-	3
10369	-	-	-	-	-	-	-	-	-	-	-	-	-	-	-	4
11730	-	-	-	-	-	-	-	-	-	-	-	-	-	-	-	11
7719	-	-	-	-	-	-	-	-	-	-	-	-	-	7	-	-
6100	-	-	17	-	-	-	-	-	-	-	-	-	-	-	-	-
7310	-	-	-	-	-	-	-	-	-	-	-	-	-	-	14	-

ID	DR	DA	DR10	DA10	GR	GA	GR10	GA10	OR	OA	OR10	OA10	PR	PA	PR10	PA10
5803	-	-	-	-	-	-	-	-	-	-	-	-	-	-	17	-
9840	-	-	-	-	-	-	-	-	-	-	-	-	-	-	-	12
6707	-	-	-	10	-	-	11	-	-	-	-	8	-	-	-	-
9861	-	-	-	-	-	-	-	-	-	-	-	-	-	-	-	13
7326	-	-	-	-	-	-	13	8	-	-	-	12	-	-	-	-
9249	-	-	-	-	-	-	-	-	-	-	-	-	-	-	-	2
8382	-	-	-	-	-	-	-	-	-	-	-	-	-	-	-	17
5561	-	-	-	3	-	-	-	3	-	-	-	3	-	-	2	-
6135	-	-	-	-	-	-	-	-	-	-	-	5	-	-	8	-
5328	-	20	-	-	-	20	-	-	-	-	-	-	-	-	-	-
6998	-	-	-	-	-	-	-	-	-	-	19	-	-	-	-	-
6620	-	-	12	13	-	-	14	12	13	13	13	11	12	-	12	-
7002	-	-	-	-	-	-	-	11	-	-	-	13	-	-	-	-
8420	-	-	-	-	-	-	-	-	-	-	-	-	-	-	-	20
5488	-	-	-	-	-	-	-	-	-	-	-	20	-	-	-	-
8847	-	-	-	7	-	-	-	-	-	-	-	-	-	-	-	-
8444	-	-	-	18	-	-	-	20	-	-	-	14	-	-	20	-
7791	-	-	-	19	-	-	-	-	-	-	-	-	-	-	-	-
9386	-	-	-	-	-	-	-	-	-	-	-	-	-	20	19	-
7174	-	-	-	14	-	-	-	15	-	-	-	-	-	-	-	-
6844	-	-	-	-	-	-	-	-	-	-	-	-	-	-	-	1
6533	-	-	-	-	-	-	-	-	-	-	-	-	-	-	-	18
2939	-	-	-	-	9	-	-	-	9	9	-	-	-	17	-	-
5349	-	-	-	4	-	-	-	4	-	-	-	4	-	-	4	-
6874	-	-	-	-	-	-	-	-	-	-	11	-	-	-	-	-
7594	-	-	-	-	-	-	-	-	-	-	-	-	-	-	-	10
6636	-	-	-	-	-	-	3	-	-	-	-	-	-	-	-	-
6544	-	-	-	-	-	-	16	-	-	-	-	-	-	-	-	19
5510	-	-	-	8	-	-	-	5	-	-	-	6	-	-	5	-
6640	-	-	-	-	-	-	15	-	-	-	-	-	-	-	-	-
6261	-	-	-	2	-	-	-	2	-	-	-	2	-	-	3	-
4938	-	-	-	-	-	-	-	-	-	-	-	-	-	-	-	-
8153	-	-	-	-	-	-	-	-	-	-	-	-	-	-	-	16
12096	-	-	-	-	-	-	-	-	-	-	-	-	-	-	-	14
11392	-	-	-	-	-	-	-	-	-	-	-	-	16	15	6

Table 9.1: Top 20 gene contributor ranking of all dogs found in reference and affected populations over 10 generations and the overall database with prob_orig.exe DR=DCM reference all dogs, DA=DCM affected all dogs, DR10=DCM reference 10 generations, DA10=DCM affected 10 generations; GR=GDV reference all dogs, GA=GDV affected all dogs, GR10=GDV reference 10 generations, GA10=GDV affected 10 generations; OR=OS reference all dogs, OA=OS affected all dogs, OR10=OS reference 10 generations, OA10=OS affected 10 generations; PR=PSS reference all dogs, PA=PSS affected all dogs, PR10=PSS reference 10 generations, PA10=PSS affected 10 generations

Right censored data ('cohort bias') in veterinary life span studies

S. R. URFER

IT is common for veterinary life span and survival estimates to be derived purely from death data and thus grouped by time of death during analysis. This leads to an artificial decrease of the estimated life span due to right censored data ('cohort bias'). This short communication uses practical examples from the literature to emphasise the necessity of applying appropriate statistical methods (such as Kaplan-Meier estimation) to life span and survival research in veterinary medicine.

With regard to survival analysis, right censored data are defined as data from the population under consideration in which death has not yet occurred at the time of study. When the sample consists of dead animals only and is sorted by death date instead of birth date, this causes a misleading decrease in life span estimates due to the fact that a certain percentage of individuals from a birth cohort are still alive at the time of sampling and thus do not appear in the death statistics. This bias is obvious when considering birth cohorts, but becomes masked when considering death cohorts.

In order for such life span evaluations to be representative, all individuals within the birth cohorts studied must already be dead. If this is not the case, and if only data of dead individuals are available, the measured life span will be influenced by the fact that death data of the individuals who are still alive will be censored. Given that these will eventually die at an older age than the dead individuals from the same birth cohort, the estimated life span will be too low. The distribution of causes of death may also be affected.

For these reasons, statistical methods have been developed to correct right censored data in survival analyses, which are commonly applied in studies from human medicine (Kalbfleisch and Prentice 2002). The most commonly used of these methods is Kaplan-Meier estimation (also known as the 'product limit estimator'), which can be used to estimate the actual survival function of the population while taking censored data into account. In some cases, right censored data can also be corrected by eliminating individuals from the data that come from birth cohorts where a significant number of individuals can be assumed to still be alive.

TABLE 1: Statistical measures of the Irish wolfhound death data provided by Bernardi (1986), demonstrating the influence of right censored data through elimination of the censored birth cohorts*

		Dogs from	
Parameter[†]	All dogs	Uncensored birth cohorts	Censored birth cohorts
Number	577	326	251
Maximum	13·50	13·50	10·00
95 per cent dead	10·42	11·25	8·88
3rd quartile	8·25	9·23	7·04
Median	6·58	7·46	5·42
1st quartile	4·83	6·00	3·75
5 per cent dead	1·73	3·17	0·96
Minimum	0·50	0·75	0·50
Mean (sd)	6·47 (2·62)	7·37 (2·47)	5·31 (2·34)

* Dogs from uncensored birth cohorts died at a significantly older age than dogs from censored birth cohorts (P<0·0001, R²=0·15, F=102·94, type III sum of squares).
† Ages are given in years

However, veterinary life span studies commonly analyse a population of dead animals (for example, coming from animal cemetery records, clinical databases or postmortem examination records) and simply use their ages at death to calculate a survival function as well as other statistical parameters regarding life span. Given that data from such sources are usually sorted by time of death rather than time of birth, right censored data are masked by this approach.

If, for example, the average life expectancy of a hypothetical group of dogs was calculated by taking the population of individuals who died in the year 2004 as the sample, the result would be too low due to right censored data. For instance, no members of the 2000 birth cohort would be recorded to have reached over four years of age. Obviously, this result does not imply that the maximum life expectancy for this cohort is four years. However, this fact becomes masked when considering these individuals as members of a death cohort.

Fig 1a shows the distributions of age at death grouped by year of birth for individuals from a study of 577 Irish Wolfhound dogs that died between 1966 and 1986 (Bernardi 1986). The original data were made available for re-analysis during the present study.

Statistical analysis of the data provided by Bernardi (1986) was carried out using linear regression by the general linear model procedure in the SAS System, version 8.02, program package. Fig 1 was created using the BOXPLOT procedure from the same package. Differences in measured life span by birth cohort due to right censored data are presented. Measured age at death is significantly different between birth cohorts (P<0·0001, R²=0·25, F=63·25, type III sum of squares [SS]). However, as Fig 1b demonstrates, when year of death is used as the grouping criterion, this bias becomes masked (P=0·09, R²=0·008, F=2·41, type III SS).

Given that very few Irish wolfhounds die aged over 12 years (Urfer and others 2007), it is possible to remove right censored data from this sample by simply removing all dogs that were born less than 12 years before the end of the data collection period. A comparison of statistical parameters before and after this removal is provided in Table 1.

During work on a review paper on life span and causes of death in Irish Wolfhounds (Urfer and others 2007), a number of articles affected by this bias in one way or another were identified in the veterinary and biological literature (Bronson 1981, 1982, Bernardi 1986, Hayashidani and others 1988, 1989, Deeb and Wolf 1994, Eichelberg and Seine 1996, Li and others 1996, Patronek and others 1997, Michell 1999, Proschowsky and others 2003, Casal and others 2006, Galis and others 2006). Their common denominator is that life

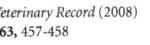

Veterinary Record (2008) 63, 457-458

S. R. Urfer, BS, DVM, Division of Animal Housing and Welfare, Vetsuisse Facility, University of Berne, Switzerland

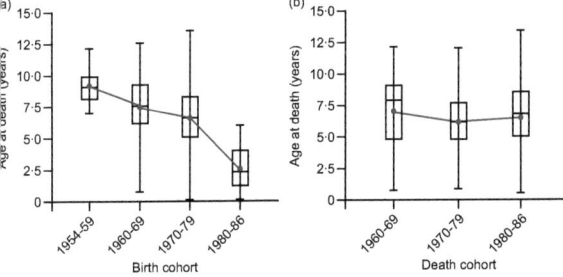

FIG 1: Death data of Irish wolfhounds used in Bernardi (1986). Dogs are grouped by (a) birth cohorts, and (b) death cohorts, as is common in life span studies

span and survival were calculated purely from death data and grouped by death cohorts, without giving due concern to the problem of right censored data.

While several possibilities for bias in veterinary life span research have already been mentioned in the literature (Reid and Peterson 2000), the problem of right censored death data has not been addressed. Life span and survival calculations based on death cohorts are widespread throughout the scientific literature. In species with long life expectancy (such as humans), this problem is particularly relevant, but its effects will be encountered whenever a significant percentage of individuals in a study come from birth cohorts of which members are still alive. In human medicine, statistical methods to correct right-censored data are commonly employed (Kalbfleisch and Prentice 2002).

In order for cohort bias due to right censored data to be eliminated from life span and survival data, populations should be analysed in cohorts grouped by their year of birth. To arrive at representative life span estimates, it is necessary to apply appropriate statistical methods to data from birth cohorts of which an important number of individuals are still alive at the time of data collection.

The data used in veterinary life span studies can be subject to some limitations – for example, grouping in very large age categories, which occurs in the Veterinary Medical Database, or lack of information on the maximum life span in the studied population. Nevertheless, the problem of right-censored data should be considered whenever a sample of life span data is analysed in veterinary science.

Using Kaplan-Meier estimation is one possible solution to the problem. In some cases, right-censored data can also be corrected sufficiently well by eliminating individuals from the data that come from birth cohorts where a significant number of individuals can be assumed to still be alive. This approach is not mathematically complex; however, depending on the structure of the studied data, it can potentially lead to the loss of an important part of the database and thus diminish the overall power of the analysis.

Given that the domestic dog is a useful model organism for life span and aging research (Austad 1993, Patronek and others 1997, Greer and others 2007), the bias caused by right-censored data deserves more consideration in veterinary and biological life span and survival studies.

ACKNOWLEDGEMENTS

The author would like to thank Sabine and Martin Gebhardt for their suggestions and critique, and Mrs Gretchen Bernardi for supplying the original data of her life span study. The work as a result of which this paper was written was partially funded by the Veterinary Competence Centre of the Swiss Army.

References

AUSTAD, S. N. (1993) FRAR course on laboratory approaches to aging. The comparative perspective and choice of animal models in aging research. *Aging (Milano)* **5**, 259-267

BERNARDI, G. (1986) Longevity and morbidity in the Irish Wolfhound in the United States – 1966 to 1986. *AKC Gazette* **105**, 70-78

BRONSON, R. T. (1981) Age at death of necropsied intact and neutered cats. *American Journal of Veterinary Research* **42**, 1606-1608

BRONSON, R. T. (1982) Variation in age at death of dogs of different sexes and breeds. *American Journal of Veterinary Research* **43**, 2057-2059

CASAL, M. L., MUNUVE, R. M., JANIS, M. A., WERNER, P. & HENTHORN, P. S. (2006) Epilepsy in Irish Wolfhounds. *Journal of Veterinary Internal Medicine* **20**, 131-135

DEEB, B. & WOLF, N. (1994) Studying longevity and morbidity in giant and small breeds of dogs. *Veterinary Medicine* **89**, 702-713

EICHELBERG, H. & SEINE, R. (1996) Life expectancy and cause of death in dogs. I. The situation in mixed breeds and various dog breeds. *Berliner und Münchener Tierärztliche Wochenschrift* **109**, 292-303 (In German)

GALIS, F., VAN DER SLUIJS, I., VAN DOOREN, T. J., METZ, J. A. & NUSSBAUMER, M. (2006) Do large dogs die young? *Journal of Experimental Zoology. B* **308**, 119-126

GREER, K. A., CANTERBERRY, S. C. & MURPHY, K. E. (2007) Statistical analysis regarding the effects of height and weight on life span of the domestic dog. *Research in Veterinary Science* **82**, 208-214

HAYASHIDANI, H., OMI, Y., OGAWA, M. & FUKUTOMI, K. (1988) Epidemiological studies on the expectation of life for dogs computed from animal cemetery records. *Nippon Juigaku Zasshi* **50**, 1003-1008

HAYASHIDANI, H., OMI, Y., OGAWA, M. & FUKUTOMI, K. (1989) Epidemiological studies on the expectation of life for cats computed from animal cemetery records. *Nippon Juigaku Zasshi* **51**, 905-908

KALBFLEISCH, J. D. & PRENTICE, R. L. (2002) The Statistical Analysis of Failure Time Data. 2nd edn. Hoboken, Wiley-Interscience

LI, Y., DEEB, B., PENDERGRASS, W. & WOLF, N. (1996) Cellular proliferative capacity and life span in small and large dogs. *Journal of Gerontology. A* **51**, B403-408

MICHELL, A. R. (1999) Longevity of British breeds of dog and its relationships with sex, size, cardiovascular variables and disease. *Veterinary Record* **145**, 625-629

PATRONEK, G. J., WATERS, D. J. & GLICKMAN, L. T. (1997) Comparative longevity of pet dogs and humans: implications for gerontology research. *Journal of Gerontology. A* **52**, B171-178

PROSCHOWSKY, H. F., RUGBJERG, H. & ERSBØLL, A. K. (2003) Mortality of purebred and mixed-breed dogs in Denmark. *Preventive Veterinary Medicine* **58**, 63-74

REID, S. W. & PETERSON, M. M. (2000) Methods of estimating canine longevity. *Veterinary Record* **147**, 630-631

URFER, S., GAILLARD, C. & STEIGER, A. (2007) Lifespan and disease predispositions in the Irish wolfhound: a review. *Veterinary Quarterly* **29**, 102-111

Acta Veterinaria Scandinavica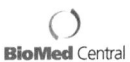

Research

Open Access

Inbreeding and fertility in Irish Wolfhounds in Sweden: 1976 to 2007
Silvan R Urfer

Address: University of Washington Medicine Pathology, 1959 NE Pacific Street, Mailbox 357470, Seattle, Washington 98195, USA
Email: Silvan R Urfer - urfer@gmx.ch

Published: 6 May 2009

Acta Veterinaria Scandinavica 2009, **51**:21 doi:10.1186/1751-0147-51-21

This article is available from: http://www.actavetscand.com/content/51/1/21

Received: 15 October 2008
Accepted: 6 May 2009

© 2009 Urfer; licensee BioMed Central Ltd.
This is an Open Access article distributed under the terms of the Creative Commons Attribution License (http://creativecommons.org/licenses/by/2.0), which permits unrestricted use, distribution, and reproduction in any medium, provided the original work is properly cited.

Abstract

Background: Given that no influence of inbreeding on life expectancy could be demonstrated in Irish Wolfhounds in a previous study, it was decided to test the influence of inbreeding and other parameters on fertility in this breed.

Methods: The study was based on all Irish Wolfhound litters registered in Sweden between 1976 and 2007 (n = 822 litters) as provided by the Swedish Kennel Club (SKK) and combined with a pedigree database going back to 1862. Analyses were performed using linear regression in a Generalised Linear Model and other tests in the SAS system®.

Results: Mean number of pups per litter was 6.01 ± 2.65, with a maximum of 13. There were no significant differences in either the number of litters or the number of pups between years of birth. Males were used for breeding at a significantly earlier age than females. Mean number of litters per parent was 2.96 ± 3.14 for males and 1.59 ± 0.87 for females. No influence of Wright's inbreeding coefficients over 5, 10, 20 and 30 generations and/or Meuwissen's inbreeding coefficients on litter size was detected. In the Generalised Linear Model, highly significant, but weak (coefficient of determination (R^2) = 0.0341) influences were found for maternal age at mating as well as maternal inbreeding measured by Wright's inbreeding coefficient over 30 generations and Meuwissen's inbreeding coefficient. Paternal inbreeding coefficients over 5, 10, 20 and 30 generations and calculated after Meuwissen, as well as maternal inbreeding coefficients over 5, 10 and 20 generations did not have significant effects on litter size.

Conclusion: The low coefficient of determination (R^2) value of the Generalised Linear Model indicates that inbreeding does not have a strong influence on fertility in Irish Wolfhounds, which is consistent with earlier results and the breed's genetic history. These results likely reflect the aforementioned genetic history and should not be extrapolated to other breeds without prior breed-specific research.

Background

Modern purebred dogs have been created through selective inbreeding of desired phenotypes regarding both appearance and temperament, leading to frequent bottlenecks in population history. Therefore, inbreeding is a major concern in purebred dog populations, and detrimental effects of inbreeding on fitness and the incidence of hereditary diseases have been demonstrated in several breeds (e.g. [1-3]). There is currently a movement amongst both the scientific veterinary and the cynological communities to establish breeding programs with the goal of minimising inbreeding in purebred dogs. The underlying idea is that given that inbreeding has been shown to have detrimental effects that affect the well-being of dogs, the reduction of inbreeding coefficients is a matter of animal welfare [4,5].

From a population genetics point of view, inbreeding results in an increase in homozygosity, as well as the loss of alleles in a population. Inbreeding depression in a population can only occur if allelic effects are not strictly additive – some degree of dominant-recessive interaction is necessary. Two models explaining inbreeding depression can be currently found in the literature: The partial dominance model, which states that the depression is due to recessive deleterious alleles that occur more frequently in a homozygous genotype in inbred populations, and the overdominance model, which states that the inbreeding-associated decrease in heterozygosity has a negative effect in itself even in the absence of deleterious alleles [6]. Current research seems to favour the partial dominance model, although a contribution according to the overdominance model cannot be ruled out [7].

The partial dominance model proposes that inbreeding depression can be overcome by a mechanism called "purging of the genetic load": Given that deleterious recessive alleles occur in the homozygous configuration more commonly in inbred populations, selection for fitness tends to eradicate them from a population more effectively than it would in a non-inbred population [7]. Purging may be intensified after a population bottleneck if deleterious alleles are subject to selection [8,9].

In the case of Irish Wolfhounds, four distinct bottleneck phenomena resulted in particularly high inbreeding coefficients due to the small size of the effective breeding population during most of the breed's history before 1960, their geographically limited distribution and the influence of both World Wars, during which widespread food rationing made the keeping of large dogs difficult. It was already hypothesised in 1956 that the breed would no longer be subject to inbreeding depression due to its genetic history [10], and a more recent study found no influence of inbreeding on life expectancy in a population of over 1'400 Irish Wolfhounds with known lifespan out of a pedigree database of over 50'000 individuals [11].

Given that the veterinary literature states that inbreeding depression not only has a negative influence on general fitness, but also on fertility parameters such as litter size and periparital mortality [12,13], it was decided to further test the hypothesis of a lack of inbreeding influence in Irish Wolfhounds through analysing the relationship between inbreeding coefficients and litter size in the breed. Since influences of maternal parity and season on litter size have also been described in the dog [14], the data were also analysed for a possible influence of these variables.

Dogs, materials and methods
Dogs
The Swedish Kennel Club (SKK) has published its registration information for Irish Wolfhounds on the internet, with information on complete registered litters going back to 1976 [15]. The SKK registers all living pups from a given litter at the latest 5 months after their birth. The absolute majority of Irish Wolfhounds in Sweden are registered with the SKK. These data were thus chosen as a means of assessing inbreeding effects on fertility on the breed. This resulted in a population of n = 5'000 dogs (2'521 males, 2'479 females) originating from 832 litters.

Pedigrees were derived from the database of the SKK and merged with an existing pedigree database going back to the beginning of modern breeding in the 1860s [11]. Litters that did not have complete pedigrees available over at least 7 generations after merging were discarded, resulting in n = 4'940 dogs (2'490 males, 2'450 females) out of 822 litters.

Parameters Studied
We chose the number of registered pups per litter as our dependent variable and determined Wright's inbreeding coefficients [16] over 5, 10, 20 and 30 generations as well as Meuwissen's inbreeding coefficients [17] for every litter as well as every parent. Furthermore, we considered the year of birth of the litters and the ages of both sire and dam at the time of mating, as well as dam parity and season as possible influences on litter size in our population.

Number of registered pups per litter was defined as the number of pups that appear in the SKK registration database, in which no data on original litter size and periparital mortality are made available online. Time of mating was determined by subtracting 63 days (the average gestation period of the domestic dog) from the date of birth of a litter. Ages at mating were calculated from the dates of birth of sire and dam respectively, as provided in the registration data. All ages were measured in days for statistical analysis. One litter had resulted from artificial insemination with frozen semen from a dead male; this litter was excluded from the calculation. Seasons were defined as Spring: March to May; Summer: June to August; Autumn: September to November; Winter: December to February, as used by [14].

Software
Pedigree data were managed in Microsoft Excel® 2007 and Pedigree Explorer® version 5.4.1FC [18] and analysed in The SAS System® version 9.1.3 SP 4. Wright's inbreeding coefficients over 5, 10, 20 and 30 generations were calculated through the "Bulk COI" procedure in Pedigree Explorer, while Meuwissen's inbreeding coefficients were calculated using the meuw.exe module of the PEDIG pro-

gram package [19]. Tables and bar graphs were created in Microsoft Excel 2007, while box plots were created using PROC BOXPLOT in The SAS System®. The box plots show minimum, 25%, 50%, 75% and maximum percentiles (red lines), as well as arithmetic means (black asterisks).

Statistical Methods

Data were analysed for significant effects in a linear regression model using PROC GLM and PROC STEPWISE in The SAS System. A type III Sum of Squares (SS) Generalised Linear Model was used. Normality testing was performed using PROC UNIVARIATE in The SAS System, while other statistical tests (Chi-Square test, Wilcoxon rank sum test, ANOVA, Kruskal-Wallis test) were performed using PROC NPAR1WAY. A P = 0.05 was considered statistically significant.

Results

Population Structure

The complete data consisted of 2'521 male and 2'479 female registered Irish Wolfhound pups out of 832 registered litters. When only individuals with complete pedigree information over 7 generations were considered, the data consisted of 2'490 males and 2'450 females from 822 registered litters. Sex distribution did not significantly differ from an equal distribution model either before or after the exclusion of litters with incomplete pedigrees (χ^2 = 0.35, P = 0.55 before exclusion and χ^2 = 0.32, P = 0.57 after exclusion). The mean number of litters per sire was 2.96 ± 3.14, with a maximum of 18. The mean number of litters per dam was 1.59 ± 0.87, with a maximum of 5.

Figure 1 shows the distribution of litters and the number of registered pups in the studied data. Mean number of pups per litter was 6.01 ± 2.65, ranging from 1 to 13 pups per litter. Litter size distribution was non-normal (Shapiro-Wilk P < 0.0001; also see figure 2). Mean number of litters per year was 26.00 ± 7.02, ranging from 12 to 42. Mean number of registered pups per year was 156.25 ± 39.73, ranging from 72 to 257. Both of these variables were normally distributed (Shapiro-Wilk P = 0.61 and P = 0.77 respectively). There were no significant differences

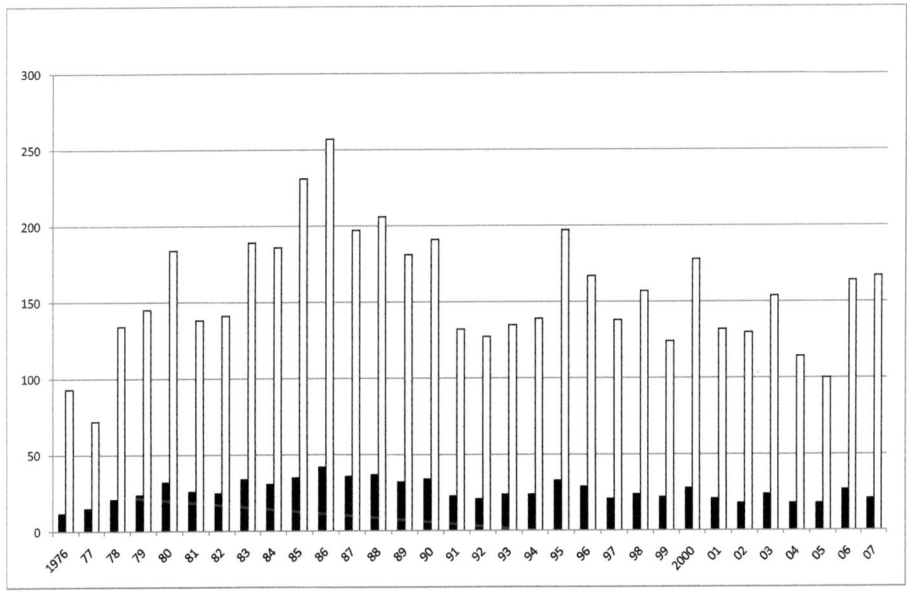

Figure 1
Registered litters and pups – 1976 to 2007. Distribution of the number of litters and the number of registered pups in the study population by year of birth. Black bars: number of litters; white bars: number of pups.

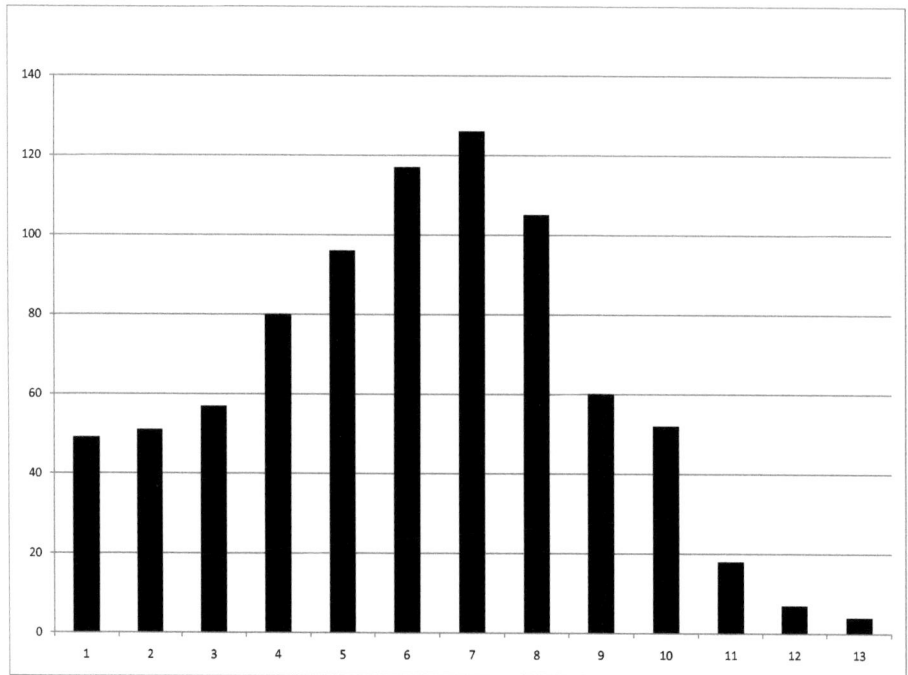

Figure 2
Distribution of litter sizes (n = 822). Distribution of litter sizes in the study population. Horizontal axis: number of pups per litter; Vertical axis: frequency of litter size. The non-normal distribution is evident.

between either the number of litters per year (P = 0.28, ANOVA) or the number of pups per year (P = 0.66, ANOVA).

Distribution of Inbreeding Coefficients

The results for Wright's inbreeding coefficients over 5, 10, 20 and 30 generations, as well as Meuwissen's inbreeding coefficients for every litter with complete pedigrees over at least 7 generations are reproduced in Table 1.

The development of inbreeding coefficients over time was also analysed graphically (see figures 3 and 4). In the Generalised Linear Model, there was a significant influence of year of birth on both Wright's inbreeding coefficient over

Table 1: Inbreeding coefficients

	Litters	Sires	Dams
5 Generations	0.0459 ± 0.0471	0.0602 ± 0.0582	0.0509 ± 0.0505
10 Generations	0.1559 ± 0.0555	0.1721 ± 0.0607	0.1621 ± 0.0575
20 Generations	0.2877 ± 0.0436	0.2859 ± 0.0495	0.2764 ± 0.0472
30 Generations	0.3290 ± 0.0397	0.3349 ± 0.0449	0.3245 ± 0.0433
Meuwissen	0.3331 ± 0.0407	0.3374 ± 0.0454	0.3267 ± 0.0439

Mean inbreeding coefficients ± Standard Deviation in the studied litters and their parents. Generational inbreeding coefficients were calculated using Wright's Method.

10 generations and Meuwissen's inbreeding coefficient, with linear regression estimates of -0.003 for Wright's inbreeding coefficient over 10 generations and +0.0015 for Meuwissen's inbreeding coefficient.

Ages at Mating, Dam Parity and Season

Mean age at mating was 1'169 ± 555 days in males and 1'396 ± 451 days in females. Ages at mating ranged from 275 to 2'948 days in males and from 512 to 2'694 days in females. This difference between the sexes was highly significant ($P < 0.0001$, two-sided Wilcoxon rank sum test). Ages at mating are rendered graphically in figure 5.

Given that it has been mentioned in the literature that male Irish Wolfhounds experience a more rapid decrease in semen quality than dogs do on average as they age [20,21], the age of the sire at mating was also tested separately for a possible influence on litter size. Our analysis did not show a significant influence, however ($P = 0.1651$, Kruskal-Wallis-Test).

Increasing maternal parity had a significant negative influence on litter size when considered by itself ($P = 0.0241$, Kruskal-Wallis test), but not when considered as part of the Generalised Linear Model. Results are rendered in table 2.

There were highly significant differences between the number of litters per season ($\chi^2 = 24.34$, $P < 0.0001$), with the most litters being born during Spring (n = 256) and the least litters being born during Autumn (n = 156). However, no influence of season on litter size could be detected ($P = 0.6634$, Kruskal-Wallis test). Results are rendered in table 3.

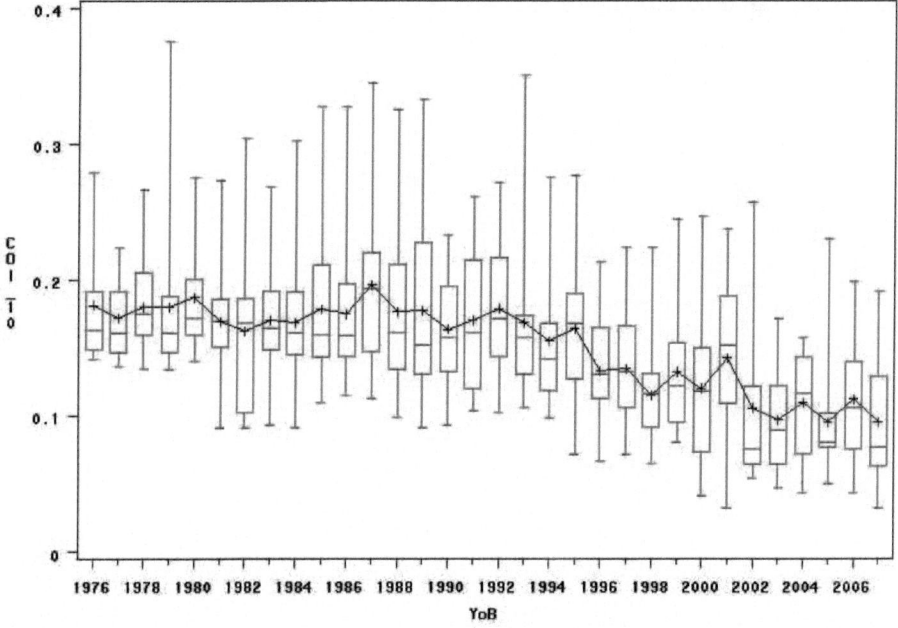

Figure 3
Inbreeding over time – 10 generations. Variations in inbreeding coefficients over time, calculated following Wright's method over 10 generations. YoB = Year of Birth; COI_10 = Wright's Inbreeding Coefficient over 10 Generations.

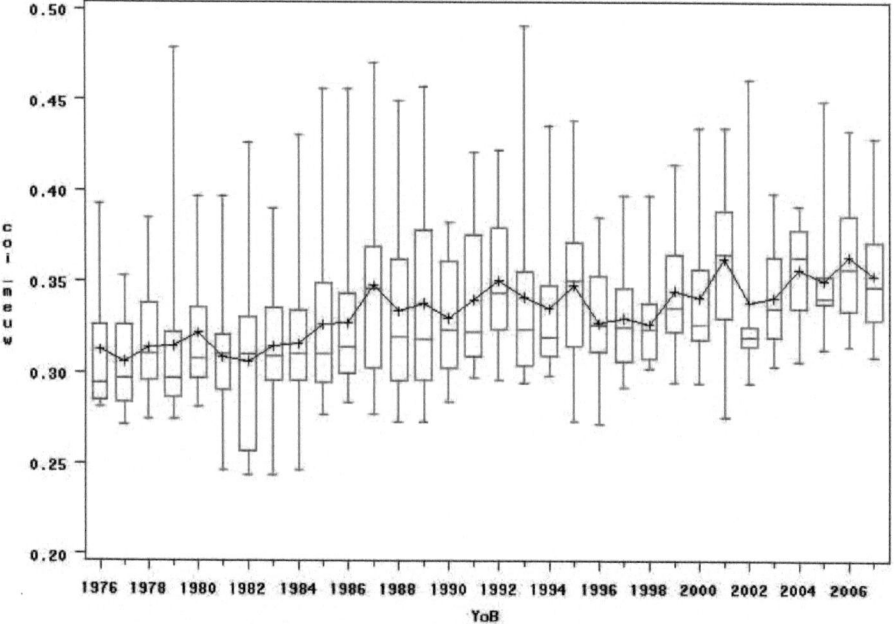

Figure 4
Inbreeding over time – Meuwissen. Variations in inbreeding coefficients over time, calculated following Meuwissen's method back to the beginning of the pedigree database. YoB = Year of Birth; COI_meuw = Meuwissen's Inbreeding Coefficient. Note the scale difference in the vertical axes between figg. 3 and 4.

Linear Regression
Based on the variables enumerated above, linear regression was performed with the goal of constructing a model that best explained the observed variance in registered litter size. Given that normality testing showed non-normal distributions for all studied independent variables, which could not be corrected through log-transformation, a type III Sum of Squares generalised linear model (GLM) was used to establish the influence of different parameters on litter size. This resulted in significant influences of the age of the dam at mating, as well as maternal inbreeding over 30 generations and after Meuwissen; however, the coefficient of determination of the model was low (R^2 = 0.0341). The other variables mentioned previously did not have a significant influence on litter size in any of the models. Results are rendered in table 4 and figures 6, 7 and 8. Results for the Generalised Linear Model including all parameters are rendered in table 5.

Discussion
While we did not find a significant effect of either a litter's own or its sire's inbreeding coefficients on registered litter size, our results demonstrate a highly significant influence of both maternal age and maternal inbreeding. However, the coefficient of determination (R^2) of the model is low, indicating that the numeric influence of these factors is low despite their high significance. This result, combined with the fact that no influence of other inbreeding parameters (e.g. inbreeding coefficients of the litter itself and its sire) on registered litter size could be found, would seem to confirm the hypothesis that inbreeding does not have an important influence on fertility in Irish Wolfhounds.

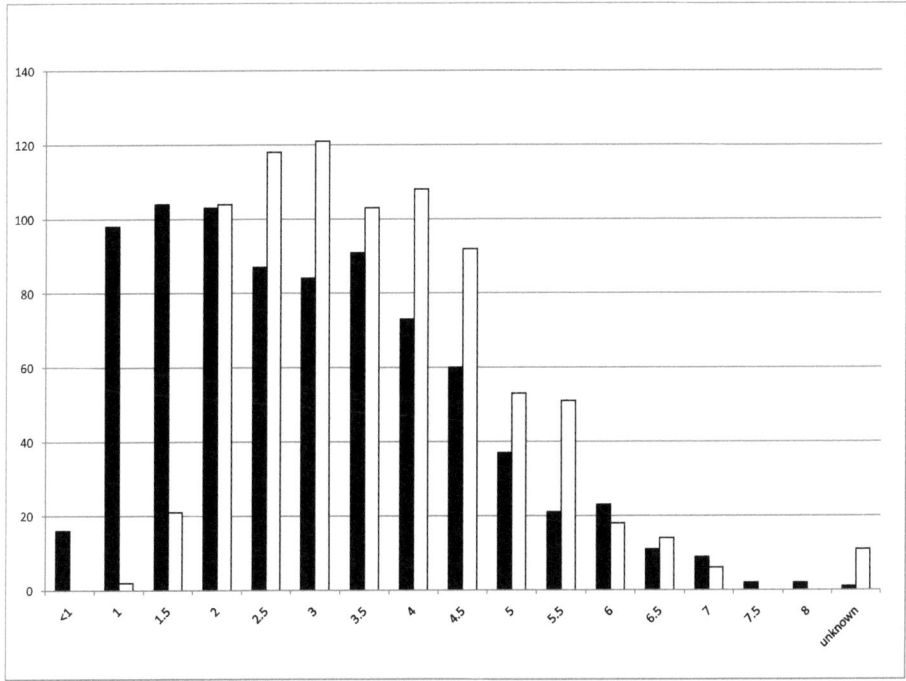

Figure 5
Ages at mating. Distribution of ages at mating in males (black) and females (white). Horizontal axis: age in years; vertical axis: number of individuals.

In practice, one might call the choice of the numbers of generations used to calculate the inbreeding coefficients arbitrary (5, 10, 20, 30 generations and Meuwissen's coefficient going back to the beginning of the data). The number of considered inbreeding coefficients was kept at this level out of both practical and statistical considerations: Wright's inbreeding coefficients above 20 generations are cumbersome and time-intensive to calculate using our software, and including every possible inbreeding coefficient between two and thirty generations would have raised the risk of false positives above an acceptable level. When also considering the fact that inbreeding coefficients over different numbers of generations are not independent, testing inbreeding over every possible number of generations thus seems unnecessary.

Table 2: Maternal parity and litter size

Parity	N	Mean Litter Size	SD
1	514	6.13	2.60
2	210	6.08	2.83
3	66	5.26	2.46
4	27	5.26	2.41
5	5	4.40	2.51

Maternal parity and litter size. N = number of litters; SD = Standard Deviation.

Table 3: Number of litters per season

Season	Litters
Spring	256
Summer	205
Autumn	156
Winter	205

Number of litters per season. Spring = March to May; Summer = June to August; Autumn = September to November; Winter = December to February.

Table 4: Multiple linear regression I

	F Value	P Value
Model	9.43	< 0.0001
Age of Dam	12.28	0.0005
Dam Inbreeding (30)	14.95	0.0001
Dam Inbreeding (Meuw)	14.71	0.0001

Generalised Linear Model (GLM type III Sum of Squares) of the significant parameters in our data and their influence on litter size. There are three degrees of freedom; the model has a coefficient of determination of $R^2 = 0.0341$.

The change in inbreeding coefficients shown in figures 3 and 4 seems striking when comparing Wright's coefficient over 10 generations and Meuwissen's coefficient. However, at least some of the decrease over 10 generations is artificial and can be explained through the exponential growth of the Irish Wolfhound breeding population that can be observed since the 1960's [11], while inbreeding coefficients calculated back to the onset of modern breeding keep increasing. Nevertheless, the fact that high inbreeding coefficients in dogs have been criticised by veterinary geneticists more recently may also have played a certain role in the recent decrease in Wright's inbreeding coefficients by motivating breeders to selectively use breeding combinations with lower inbreeding coefficients over a lower number of generations.

Table 5: Multiple linear regression II

	F Value	P Value
Model	2.17	0.0010
COI 5	0.03	0.8705
COI 10	0.21	0.6487
COI 20	1.84	0.1752
COI 30	2.93	0.0873
COI meuw	2.46	0.1172
pat COI 5	1.19	0.2765
pat COI 10	0.00	0.9785
pat COI 20	0.95	0.3291
pat COI 30	2.87	0.0906
pat COI meuw	2.46	0.1171
mat COI 5	3.00	0.0838
mat COI 10	1.29	0.2570
mat COI 20	0.14	0.7113
mat COI 30	5.46	0.0197
mat COI meuw	6.99	0.0084
Parity	1.21	0.3047
Season	0.58	0.6288
Age of sire at mating	3.45	0.0637
Age of dam at mating	5.88	0.0155

Generalised Linear Model (GLM type III Sum of Squares) of all parameters in our data and their influence on litter size. There are 24 degrees of freedom; the model has a coefficient of determination of $R^2 = 0.0627$. COI 5, 10, 20, 30, meuw refer to the inbreeding coefficients of the litter, pat COI to the inbreeding coefficients of the sire, mat COI to the inbreeding coefficients of the dam.

The study at hand is based on a database of registered pups. The studied data did not include information on how many pups in these litters died before the litters were registered, and consequently, there is no way of assessing peripartal mortality as a possible consequence of inbreeding in the data. Furthermore, the present data do not provide any means of assessing the percentage of fertile versus infertile matings. Such data are not made available online. However, the SKK litter registration forms contain fields for original litter size and peripartal mortality, and these data could be used in future research to determine whether or nor they are influenced by inbreeding.

The geographical scope of this study is limited to litters bred and registered in Sweden, which may lead to concerns of the data not being representative for the Irish Wolfhound breed in general. However, previous research has demonstrated that all Irish Wolfhounds alive worldwide during the study time can be traced back to one recent bottleneck in the 1950's [11].

The data showed a significant negative influence of maternal parity on litter size when parity was considered by itself, but this influence did not remain significant when considered as part of the Generalised Linear Model. Given that an influence of maternal parity on litter size has been described previously [14], it was decided to nevertheless include these results separately in table 2.

As opposed to reference [14], which described a significantly larger litter size for litters born during Spring, we did not find any seasonal influence on litter size, but found that a significantly increased number of litters had been born during Spring. The difference in the number of litters per season may reflect a possible influence of season on the females' sexual cycle rather than a change in other fertility parameters, which could be expected to result in seasonal changes in litter size. However, it is also possible that the Swedish breeders are planning their litters in a way that will make rearing the pups more convenient, which would seem to be easier with a litter whelped in Spring than with one whelped during Autumn due to climatic considerations.

When comparing the present results to the results of [14], however, it should be noted that the latter only found an influence of season on litter size when considering one privately owned commercial kennel, but not when considering the whole SKK database, and concluded from this that the wide variation in husbandry practices between different breeders would obscure any such influence in a large multi-kennel database. If this interpretation is correct, the same would apply to the results of the study at hand, and it is thus possible that significant seasonal

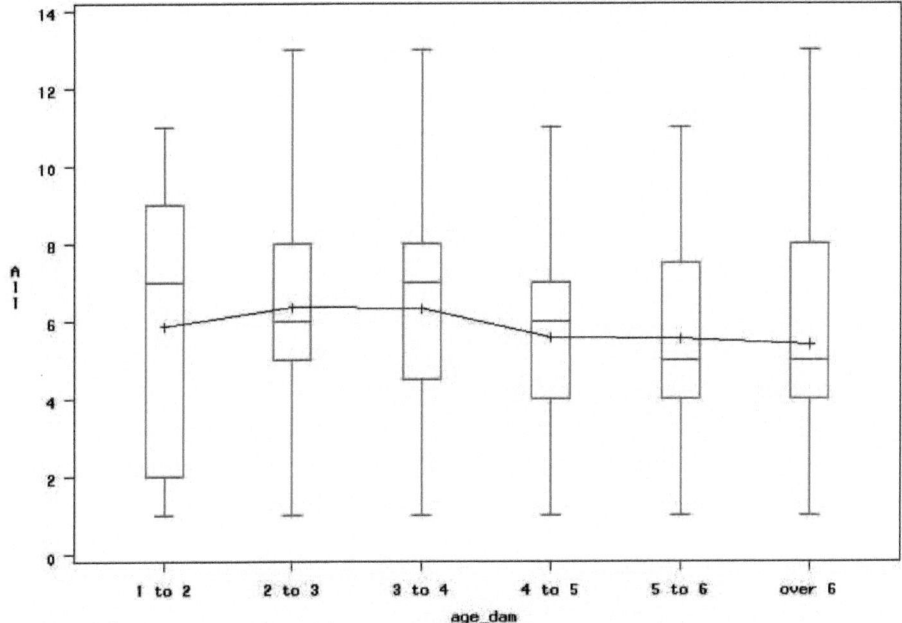

Figure 6
Age of dam at mating and litter size. Maternal age at mating and registered litter size. All: registered litter size; age_dam: maternal age at mating (years). Graphical rendering of significant effects in table 4. Although these effects are highly significant, actual influence on litter size remains low, as expressed by the low coefficient of determination ($R^2 = 0.0341$).

effects on litter size could also exist in individual Irish Wolfhound kennels.

The relatively low average breeding age of the females in the present population can only be partially explained by the breed's comparably low life expectancy and the fact that SKK regulations generally prohibit the use of Irish Wolfhound bitches above seven years of age for breeding. It seems that in addition to these circumstances, Swedish Irish Wolfhound breeders are generally reluctant to use their bitches for breeding at a more advanced age due to their perception that this results in a higher risk of potentially deadly complications (Blom, personal communication).

Using males for breeding at a comparably young age also seems to be commonplace in the study population. This may be due to the fact that procreation tends to be less of a burden on their organism than it is in females, but may also be influenced by previous findings that male Irish Wolfhounds experience a marked decrease in semen quality and libido at a younger age than average dogs [20,21]. This could motivate the breeders to use their males at a young age, and it could also distort the influence of older males on the number of registered litters by increasing the percentage of failed matings when older males are used. While our results do not show an influence of paternal age on litter size in either the generalised linear model or the individual Kruskal-Wallis statistical test, the previously published age-related decrease in libido could also have influenced this age distribution.

Conclusions

In view of the very low coefficient of determination (R^2) of the Generalised Linear Model, the present data support the hypothesis that inbreeding does not play an impor-

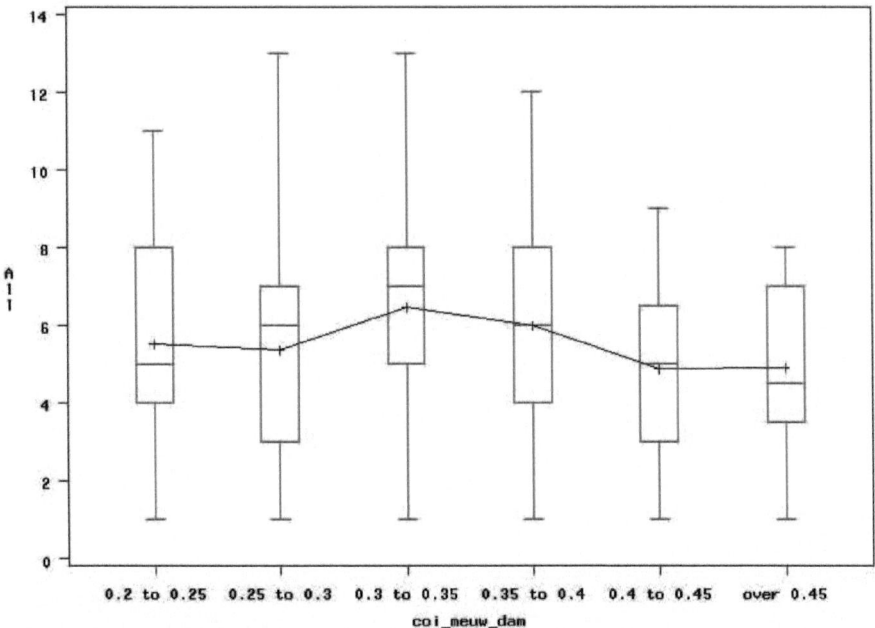

Figure 7
COI (Meuw) of dam and litter size. Maternal Meuwissen's inbreeding coefficient and registered litter size. All: registered litter size; coi_meuw_dam: maternal Meuwissen's inbreeding coefficient. Graphical rendering of significant effects in table 4. Although these effects are highly significant, actual influence on litter size remains low, as expressed by the low coefficient of determination (R^2 = 0.0341).

tant role among factors determining fertility in Irish Wolfhounds. More research is required to determine whether there is an inbreeding influence on fertile versus infertile matings and peripartal mortality in the breed.

In dog breeding, it is highly unusual to have data on 30 and more generation as a basis of inbreeding calculation. Therefore, and also considering the low coefficient of determination (R^2) value of the present model, it seems unlikely that this study's findings concerning the influence of maternal inbreeding coefficients and age on registered litter size will play an important role in future Irish Wolfhound breeding practices.

The author would like to stress out that these results likely reflect the unique genetic history of Irish Wolfhounds as a breed and should not be generalised to apply to breeds in which a detrimental effect of inbreeding has been clearly demonstrated. Most breeds would not have been subject to as severe bottleneck events during their recent genetic history as Irish Wolfhounds have [11], and even in breeds that have gone through comparable bottleneck events, the elimination of inbreeding depression through purging following such events is one possible consequence, but by no means an obligatory occurrence [8,9]. Therefore, the application of the present findings to other breeds should not be attempted without first analysing similar data from these breeds.

Competing interests
The author declares that they have no competing interests.

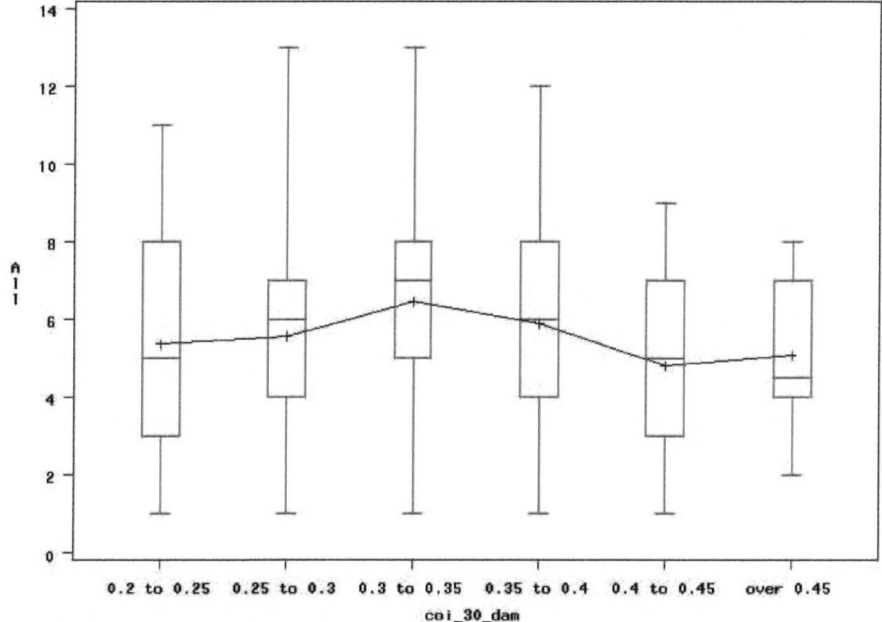

Figure 8
COI (30) of dam and litter size. Maternal Wright's inbreeding coefficient over 30 generations and litter size. All: registered litter size; coi_30_dam: maternal Wright's inbreeding coefficient over 30 generations. Graphical rendering of significant effects in table 4. Although these effects are highly significant, actual influence on litter size remains low, as expressed by the low coefficient of determination (R^2 = 0.0341).

Acknowledgements
The author would like to thank Prof. Anna Blom, PhD, of Lund University for her suggestions concerning the use of the SKK data, as well as her critique; Ms. Amy André, BS, for her invaluable help with the original pedigree database; as well as Ms. A.I. Gottsch of the Irish Wolfhound Research Database [22], for filling in various gaps in the pedigree information.

This study was funded by the Swiss National Science Foundation http://www.snf.ch, project-N° PBBEB-119243.

References
1. Beek S van der, Nielen AL, Schukken YH, Brascamp EW: **Evaluation of genetic, common-litter, and within-litter effects on preweaning mortality in a birth cohort of puppies.** Am J Vet Res 1999, **60:**1106-1110.
2. Gresky C, Hamann H, Distl O: **[Influence of inbreeding on litter size and the proportion of stillborn puppies in dachshunds].** Volume 118. Berl Munch Tierarztl Wochenschr; 2005:134-139.
3. Boenigk K, Hamann H, Distl O: **[Genetic-statistical analysis of environmental and genetic influences on the outcome of the juvenile and breeding performance tests for behaviour traits in Hovawart dogs].** Berl Munch Tierarztl Wochenschr 2006, 119:258-269.
4. Arman K: **A new direction for kennel club regulations and breed standards.** Can Vet J 2007, **48:**953-965.
5. Wachtel H: **Hundezucht 2000 [Dog Breeding 2000].** 3rd edition. Germany: Kynos; 2007.
6. Charlesworth D, Charlesworth B: **Inbreeding Depression and its Evolutionary Consequences.** Annu Rev Ecol Syst 1987, 18:237-268.
7. Crnokrak P, Barrett SC: **Perspective: purging the genetic load: a review of the experimental evidence.** Evolution. 2002, 56(12):2347-2358.
8. Fowler K, Whitlock MC: **The variance in inbreeding depression and the recovery of fitness in bottlenecked populations.** Proc Biol Sci 1999, **266:**2061-2066.
9. Kirkpatrick M, Jarne P: **The Effects of a Bottleneck on Inbreeding Depression and the Genetic Load.** Am Nat 2000, **155:**154-167.
10. Comfort A: **Longevity and Mortality of Irish Wolfhounds.** Proc Zoolog Soc London 1956, **CXXVII:**27-34.
11. Urfer SR: **Lifespan and Causes of Death in Irish Wolfhounds: Medical, Genetical and Ethical Aspects.** DVM Thesis 2007 [http:/

[/www.ths.vetsuisse.unibe.ch/lenya/housing/live/publications/Diss_Urfer_2007.pdf]. University of Berne, Institute of Animal Genetics, Nutrition and Housing, Vetsuisse Faculty
12. Wildt DE, Baas EJ, Chakraborty PK, Wolfle TL, Stewart AP: **Influence of inbreeding on reproductive performance, ejaculate quality and testicular volume in the dog.** *Theriogenology* 1982, **17:**445-452.
13. Peyer N: **[Assessing breeding-related defects in purebred dogs for their relevance in animal protection] (Die Beurteilung zuchtbedingter Defekte bei Rassehunden in tierschützerischer Hinsicht).** In *DVM Thesis* University of Bern, DVM Thesis; 1997.
14. Gavrilovic BB, Andersson K, Linde Forsberg C: **Reproductive patterns in the domestic dog – a retrospective study of the Drever breed.** *Theriogenology* 2008, **70:**783-794.
15. Anonymous: **SKK HUNDDATA.** *Svenska kennelklubben* 2008 [http://kennet.skk.se/hunddata/].
16. Wright S: **Coefficients of Inbreeding and Relationship.** *The American Naturalist* 1922, **56:**330.
17. Meuwissen THE, Luo Z: **Computing inbreeding coefficients in large populations.** *Genet Sel Evol* 1992, **24:**305-313.
18. de Jong R: **Pedigree Explorer – program for the management of pedigree data.** 5.4.1 edition. 2002 [http://www.breedmate.com].
19. Boichard D, Maignel L, Verrier E: **The value of using probabilities of gene origins to measure genetic variability in a population.** *Genet Sel Evol* 1997, **29:**5-23.
20. Dahlbom M, Andersson M, Huszenicza G, Alanko M: **Poor semen quality in Irish wolfhounds: a clinical, hormonal and spermatological study.** *J Small Anim Pract* 1995, **36:**547-552.
21. Dahlbom M, Andersson M, Juga J, Alanko M: **Fertility parameters in male Irish wolfhounds: a two-year follow-up study.** *J Small Anim Pract* 1997, **38:**547-550.
22. **The Irish Wolfhound Research Database** [http://www.ianinas.com/pedigree.html]

Publish with **BioMed Central** and every scientist can read your work free of charge

"BioMed Central will be the most significant development for disseminating the results of biomedical research in our lifetime."
Sir Paul Nurse, Cancer Research UK

Your research papers will be:

- available free of charge to the entire biomedical community
- peer reviewed and published immediately upon acceptance
- cited in PubMed and archived on PubMed Central
- yours — you keep the copyright

Submit your manuscript here:
http://www.biomedcentral.com/info/publishing_adv.asp

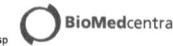

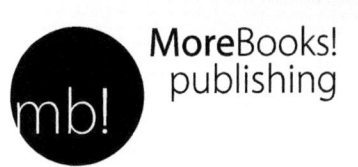

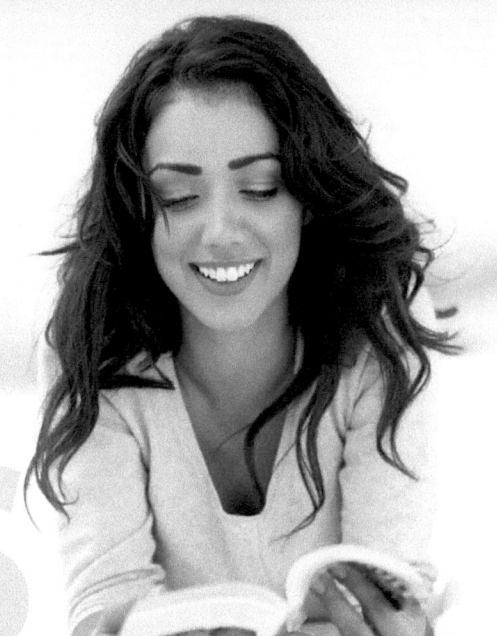

i want morebooks!

Buy your books fast and straightforward online - at one of world's fastest growing online book stores! Environmentally sound due to Print-on-Demand technologies.

Buy your books online at
www.get-morebooks.com

Kaufen Sie Ihre Bücher schnell und unkompliziert online – auf einer der am schnellsten wachsenden Buchhandelsplattformen weltweit! Dank Print-On-Demand umwelt- und ressourcenschonend produziert.

Bücher schneller online kaufen
www.morebooks.de

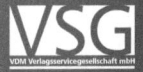

VDM Verlagsservicegesellschaft mbH
Heinrich-Böcking-Str. 6-8　　Telefon: +49 681 3720 174　　info@vdm-vsg.de
D - 66121 Saarbrücken　　　Telefax: +49 681 3720 1749　　www.vdm-vsg.de

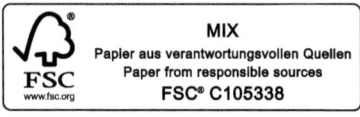

Printed by Books on Demand GmbH, Norderstedt / Germany